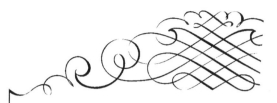
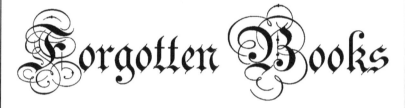
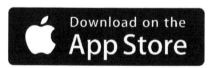
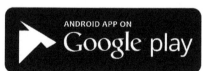

ISBN 978-1-330-31887-4
PIBN 10025534

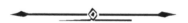

56 & 58 LAFAYETTE PLACE NE

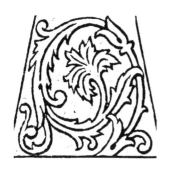

VOLUME 3 NU

JULY 188

CONTENTS OF THE NEXT ISSUE.

VOLUME III.   NUMBER I.

WOOD'S

Medical and Surgical MONOGRAPHS

Consisting of Original Treatises and of Complete Reproductions, in English, of Books and Monographs selected from the latest literature of foreign countries, with all illustrations, etc.

CONTENTS

PUBLISHED MONTHLY

PRICE, $10.00 A YEAR   SINGLE COPIES, $1.00

JULY, 1889

NEW YORK

WILLIAM WOOD AND COMPANY

56 AND 58 LAFAYETTE PLACE

PRESS OF

THE PUBLISHERS' PRINTING COMPANY,

157-159 WILLIAM STREET,

NEW YORK.

CONTENTS.

CANCER AND CANCEROUS DISEASES.

CARDIAC DYSPNŒA AND CARDIAC ASTHMA.

THE INFLUENCE OF MENSTRUATION AND OF PATHOLOGICAL CONDITIONS OF THE UTERUS ON CUTANEOUS DISEASES.

TENSION IN SURGICAL PRACTICE. INFLAMMATION OF BONE AND CRANIAL AND INTRACRANIAL INJURIES.

LECTURE I.

CANCER

AND CANCEROUS DISEASES

BY

SIR SPENCER WELLS, Bart., F.R.C.S.

7—1

CANCER AND CANCEROUS DISEASES.

LAST year, Sir James Paget delivered for the first time the Morton Lecture on cancer and cancerous diseases. He dedicated his published lecture to Mr. John Thomas Morton, of Caterham Valley, "with sincere respect for his benevolence and generosity," and expressed the hope, which he believed Mr. Morton entertained, that this lectureship may lead to some practical utility, "perhaps even to the finding of a method for the prevention or the cure of these diseases." No body of men can be more anxious to assist in the attainment of this philanthropic desire than are the fellows and members of this college. Not one of us needs to be reminded of the almost overwhelming importance of the subject. Cancerous diseases are as heart-breaking to the surgeon as they are mysterious and terrible to the public. And additional reasons for urging the importance of their study now may be found in the fact that, notwithstanding the great advance in sanitary science and the prolongation of the average length of human life—in spite of the shortening of the duration and the lowering of the mortality of some diseases, the prevention, almost the stamping out, of others—cancerous diseases, so far from being less prevalent or less fatal, are increasing among us. The increase in the number of deaths from cancer is now, and has been for many years past, greater than the proportional increase of population. Doubts have been expressed whether this increase is real or only apparent, and due to more complete and accurate registration of the causes of death. This is such an extremely important question that I feel bound to ask for your attention for a few minutes while I lay before you some facts which may assist us in arriving at the truth. The forty-seventh annual Report of the Registrar-General of Births, Deaths, and Marriages in England was presented to Parliament in 1886. It contains returns of the deaths in 1884, and we find that the mortality from cancer was higher in that than in any previous year. We also learn that in three successive periods of ten years, from 1851 to 1880, and in the seven following years to 1887, there has been a gradual increase of mortality from cancer—an increase common to both sexes, but considerably greater in males than in females. Up to the age of twenty-five, the cancer mortality is small in both sexes, but at all age-periods after the twenty-fifth year the mortality is much higher of females than of males; and in both sexes there is a rapid rise of cancer mortality at all ages after twenty-five years. I am very unwilling to trouble you with figures, and yet the story they tell of increased and increasing mortality from cancer in England and Wales is so full of interest that I feel bound to ask you to glance at the tables before you, which I have prepared partly from published reports, and partly from information kindly supplied to me officially.

The first statement I wish to place before you is the fact that the number of deaths from cancer in England increased from 7,245 in 1861 to 17,113 in 1887. We know that the population increased largely during the same period; but, making the necessary correction for increase of population, and estimating the proportion of deaths from cancer to one million persons living, we arrive at remarkable results. This table shows the number of deaths from cancer in England to one million persons living in the last twenty-seven years, and I am able, through the kindness of Dr. Grimshaw, to compare the Irish and English returns for the last eleven years:—

Year.			England.	Year.				England.
1861	.	.	.	360	1869	.	.	.	417
1862	.	.	.	361	1870	.	.	.	424
1863	.	.	.	361	1871	.	.	.	423
1864	.	.	.	386	1872	.	.	.	436
1865	.	.	.	372	1873	.	.	.	444
1866	.	.	.	385	1874	.	.	.	461
1867	.	.	.	392	1875	.	.	.	471
1868	.	.	.	402	1876	.	.	.	473

Year.	England.	Ireland.	Year.	England.	Ireland.
1877	. .´ 488	350	1883	. . 546	400
1878	. . 503	360	1884	. . 560	390
1879	. . 502	340	1885	. . 566	390
1880	. . 514	340	1886	. . 583	410
1881	. . 520	370	1887	. . 606	430
1882	. . 532	370			

I think it hardly possible that this steady increase in twenty-six years from 360 to 606 deaths from cancer among each million persons living in England and Wales during that period can be truly attributed to any great extent to better registration. You see that in some successive years the mortality is almost exactly the same; but, on the whole, the increase is much more steady and regular than any modification is likely to have been in the views or habits of those who certify and those who register the causes of death.

And if we arrange the figures in groups of years—three, five, and seven years—from 1858 to 1887, the same steady increase is even more manifest. Here is the annual death-rate from cancer to a million persons living, from 1858 to 1887 and a comparison with Scotland for five of these periods:—

		England and Wales.	Scotland.
Three years (1858–60)	. . .	335	—
Five " (1861–65)	. . .	368	404
Five " (1866–70)	. . .	404	428
Five " (1871–75)	. . .	446	468
Five " (1876–80)	. . .	495	504
Five " (1881–85)	. . .	545	540
Two " (1886–87)	. . .	595	—

A glance at the first table shows that up to 1884 the mortality had reached 560, but was up to 606 in 1887. These are the returns of all ages. If we disregard the few deaths in the earlier years of life, and confine our attention to the deaths in persons of twenty-five years of age and upward, we may compare the period of thirty years before 1880 with the seven following years.

Here is the comparison:—

	Both Sexes.	[Males.	Females.
Thirty years (1851–80)	. 867	561	1144
Seven " (1881–87)	. 1229	895	1533

Surely this great increase in recent years, both among males and females, suggests an urgent need both for inquiry and explanation. I should remind you, before passing on, that if the English population consisted of an equal number of males and females, the annual death-rate from cancer per million of persons of both sexes, aged twenty-five years and upward, would be 1,214 instead of 1,229.

In order to compare England with Ireland, I have examined the last Report of Dr. Grimshaw, the Registrar-General for Ireland, and with his obliging assistance have prepared this table, which shows what the total deaths from cancer have been in England and Wales and Ireland in the eleven years 1877 to 1887 at all ages:—

Year.					Deaths in England and Wales.	Deaths in Ireland.
1877	.	.	.	.	. 12,061	1,873
1878	.	.	.	.	. 12,594	1,913
1879	.	.	.	.	. 12,722	1,782
1880	.	.	.	.	. 13,210	1,775
1881	.	.	.	.	. 13,542	1,909
1882	.	.	.	.	. 14,057	1,882
1883	.	.	.	.	. 14,614	1,995
1884	.	.	.	.	. 15,198	1,947
1885	.	.	.	.	. 15,560	1,925
1886	.	.	.	.	. 16,243	2,029
1887	.	.	.	.	. 17,113	2,067

On the whole, a smaller increase in eleven years in Ireland than in England and in some years a diminution in Ireland. If we inquire how this is affected by the number of the population, we find that an increase of the number of cancer deaths from 1,873 to 2,067 corresponds with a diminution in population of nearly half a million; and if we calculate the death-rate from cancer, not in persons of all ages, but in those aged twenty-five years and upward, we find that the deaths from cancer registered in Ireland during the seventeen years 1864 to 1880, are equal to an average annual rate of 676 per million of the living above twenty-five years of age; while those registered during the seven years 1881 to 1887 yielded an average rate of 873 per million. Pray observe—before 1880, 676 per million, and since 1880, 873—surely a remarkable increase, though not so great as in England.

The only years I have yet been able to compare Scotland with Ireland and England are 1883 and 1885, and the figures are—

Year.	England.	Scotland.	Ireland.
1883	546	550	400
1885	546	569	390

These figures represent the proportionate number of deaths to each million of living persons. If we ask only for the total number of deaths from cancer we find that in 1885 there were in Scotland 789 male and 1,384 female deaths—equal to 560 in each million living at all ages—slightly larger than in England, and much larger than in Ireland. In Scotland, with a population smaller by about one million than the Irish, there were some 200 more deaths from cancer. Dr. Cunynghame, in his Report to the Registrar-General for Scotland, remarks that the mortality is highest in Edinburgh and the large town districts, and the proportion varies very much; for while in Edinburgh 49 of every thousand specified deaths are from cancer—in Aberdeen there are 43; Perth, 35; Dundee, 28; Glasgow, in different districts, 21 to 19. Considering that there are large hospitals both in Glasgow and Edinburgh, the fact that deaths from cancer were in 1885 proportionately more than double in one city than in the other is a matter for careful inquiry. By referring to the table of cancer mortality in groups of years from 1861 to 1885 a comparison may be made with the English returns for part of the time—the general result agreeing pretty closely with the Scotch—and both showing a considerable excess over Ireland.

In the United States the recent increase of mortality has been as great as in England. According to Dr. Fordyce Barker, whose reputation here is as deservedly high as among his own countrymen, the mortality from cancer in the city of New York has risen from 400 to the million in 1875 to 530 to the million in 1885. Discussing this increased frequency and mortality of cancerous diseases "in those nations which are the most advanced in civilization," Dr. Barker says that in America these diseases are much less frequent in the colored than in the white race. Hence the mortality is less in the Southern than in the Northern States. "It causes the greatest proportion of deaths where there is the greatest proportion of people of advanced age—that is to say, in the New England States. Hence, in any given locality, a large proportion of deaths from cancer indicates, to a certain extent, that the locality is a healthy and long-settled one, and has a large proportion of inhabitants of advanced age." In this country, it would appear that, although the liability to death from cancer advances rapidly with age, as does the liability to death from other causes (in the words of our Registrar-General), "the characteristic feature of cancer mortality is not its increase with advance of years, for this it shares with other fatal affections, but its disproportionate increase in the middle periods of life."

The fact that these diseases destroy their victims during the most active and useful periods of life surely adds to the importance of studying their causes. When we learn more of their natural history, we shall know better how to avoid or prevent, perhaps to cure them; and we require more information, not only as to the geographical distribution of these diseases in general, as compared with the ages, sexes, and ocenpations of the populations of different areas, for a sufficient number of years; but it is of equal, perhaps of greater, importance to ascertain how they affect different organs according to locality, race, and habits. For example, cancer of the breast and of the womb may be more accurately recognized, during life and after death, than many other forms of cancer, and if increasing mortality of these seats of the disease were registered in country or any district, it could hardly be denied on the plea of erroneous diagnosis. I may mention a very remarkable fact which seems to prove that in one city at least deaths from these two forms of the disease are not increasing. The city of Frankfort-on-the-Maine is renowned for the completeness and accuracy of its statistics of population, and Hirsch says—in his valuable work on "Geographical and Historical Pathology" (translation for the New Sydenham Society, p. 508): "There has not only been no increase during the twenty-one years 1863 to 1883 in the frequency of those forms of cancer which can be most accurately diagnosed during life or after death, namely mammary and uterine cancer, but indeed a considerable decrease when we allow for the fact that the population has almost doubled during that period." The British Medical Association addressed the Registrar-

General last year, arguing that "the only means which offer a reasonable prospect of discovering how far the increase in the deaths from cancer is real or only apparent, lies in the tabulation, through a course of years, of the cancers of each part of the body separately." In support of the application for such additional returns, the Association urged that they might lead to further knowledge of the causes of the disease, and said: "Your returns have already shown that the increase is greater among men than among women; you may further discover that men of certain trades and employments are more liable than others to the disease, that cancer of certain organs is increasing, while that of all other parts of the body remains stationary, with similar information of equal, or even greater, value" (Brit. Med. Journ., Nov. 12, 1887).

The Registrar-General in his reply relied upon what he called "the great and regrettable lack of precision with which very many members of the medical profession state causes of death in their certificates," as one reason for not tabulating under any but "wide and general headings." Another plea, that he cannot entertain any proposal which would lead to the employment of additional clerks, is surely feeble. No Government could refuse some slight addition to the estimates for a really useful purpose. The opinion, as stated by Dr. Ogle, that some part of the increased mortality under the heading "Cancer" is due to "improved diagnosis and more precise statement of cause" may be quite true; but it is believed that more detailed statistical returns would assist us in determining whether these reasons account for little or for much of the increase and for how much. I can hardly doubt that the required information for England and Wales will be obtained if the Registrar-General has sufficient funds placed at his disposal by the Government. Dr. Grimshaw, the Registrar-General for Ireland, has already begun to obtain and supply the needful information. In his report for the year 1887 he has published a table which shows the deaths from cancer registered during the year, by sexes and age-periods, arranged according to the part of the body affected by the disease, so far as that information was contained in the returns. In 406 cases, the organ or part of the body affected was not stated, and it is important to note that of the 1,661 cases where the required information was given, 507 (or nearly a third) were from cancer of the stomach.   As twenty-nine other cases are returned for the pylorus, the proportion is still larger.   There were 203 (or about an eighth) from cancer of the breast; and 161 (about a tenth) from cancer of the uterus.   Next in order . follow the liver, tongue and lips, throat, intestines and rectum.

When we are able to compare such returns from Ireland with similar information from England, Wales, and Scotland, we may surely be assisted in our study of the causes and prevention of these diseases.

I am sorry that I cannot do more than ask you to glance at Mr. Haviland's interesting charts, which show how very greatly the geographical distribution of cancer and phthisis differ in Great Britain.   His writings on this subject merit your careful attention, especially those in the first volume of the " Lancet " for this year.

It would be unjust to Dr. Ogle if I were not gratefully to acknowledge the value of much that he has already done, and accept it as a proof that more will follow.. His observations on the varying mortality from cancer in the different counties of England, on the excessively high cancer mortality in London and the surrounding counties, and in many of the counties on the eastern half of the kingdom, and his cautious examination of the truth of the widely spread belief that " cancer mortality is lowest on the western side and highest on the eastern side of England," merits our hearty thanks.   If the Registrar-General have power enough, and the expenditure of his department is not stinted, there is ample ground for hope that all required information will be obtained and given.   But we must also do our own share of the work.   Complaints, not altogether unfounded, are made that the profession does not supply the necessary data for accuracy of statement.   It is said that not only country general practitioners, but men of high standing in London, and officials in our great hospitals, are very careless in the matter of filling up death certificates, and yet are angry when they cannot find the precise detailed statistics they desire to obtain.   All this is worthy of your careful consideration, and I cannot think I am wrong in the confident belief that hereafter members of our profession in all parts of the country, as well as our associations and medical societies, will assist the Government by freely giving their careful attention to the accuracy of the returns they make as to the causes of death, and will assist willingly and to the best of their power in the attainment of an object of such national importance. Although some inquirers have not yet obtained all the statistical information they want, I do not think it can be denied that—in regard especially to cancer—there are no statistics in the whole range of medical literature which can be compared, for fullness or for accuracy, with those given in our Registrar-General's last annual report. Not only are those returns founded on a far wider basis than any others, but they stand alone as the only statistics of cancer in which the necessary correction for age-distribution has been made— a correction without which all statistics as to the comparative frequency of cancer in the two sexes, or in different geographical areas, are almost valueless.

The time and attention you have given to these figures, and the inferences drawn from them, will not be lost if you are led, by the belief that cancer and cancerous diseases are increasing, to ask, Can the increase be checked? What are our duties as surgeons in relation to these diseases in general, and to their surgical treatment when different organs or parts of the body are attacked by them?

Upon the general question of the nature and causes of these diseases, of their prevention or the means of checking their increase, I can only speak in the most hasty manner—partly because I could add very little to what Sir James Paget said last year and to the concluding sentence, Mr. President, of your own Bradshaw lecture in this place. You there say, " Before we shall ever be able to answer the question, Why or how do tumors form? we must be able to solve the problem of normal growth and development, and to answer the queston, Why or how it is that these continue up to a certain point, and then suddenly cease? "

If I were to attempt to add to this, ıt would be necessary to review the progress of scientfic pathology in our own time, and to criticise what is known, or believed, or taught in our schools, of the processes which lead to the formation of new growths, especially of those growths which are in their character infltrating, spreading, invading, encroaching upon or supplanting, surrounding structures, and which may secondarily affect distant parts of the body. The problem is, how these growths take the place of normal tissues or structures, how their cellular elements appear in the interstices of normal textures, how the normal cells are altered or transformed, how the infecting cells are only misplaced and proliferating epithelium, not new elements, but imperfect or morbid epithelium which has acquired the power of infecting the neighboring cells, or of impressing upon them an epithelial type. You see in this drawing "cancer-cells" arising interstitially from connective-tissue cells which had reassumed their embryonic plastic character. This is the teaching of Virchow, and, though not easy to explain, seems to be in accordance with what the microscope shows us. These are problems which it would be hopeless to attempt to discuss in an hour. If we go a little further back, and study the whole cycle of changes from the cellular rudiments of organs and tissues, through

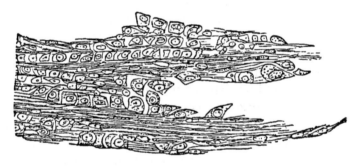

their normal growth and development toward their natural decay and death, and bear in mind the liability of some of these organs to premature obsolescence, the occasional persistence or return to embryonic forms or powers, and the risk attending the survival in the body of rudimentary structures, we open a fruitful line of inquiry. And if we combine the study of this elemental and cellular pathology with that of the changes in the blood and blood-vessels and in the nervous system modified or not by the influence of hereditary tendencies, and associated or not with the action of chemical or organic agents introduced from without, with the inoculation and multiplication of micro-organisms, and with the poisonous animal alkaloids and extractive compounds which they secrete and leave behind after their work has been done, we have a new world before us, a boundless sphere for continuous research. I know of no path of original research where more advance is to be hoped for, and none where the assistance freely offered to earnest workers in the new laboratories of this college, which are the first fruits of the bequest of Erasmus Wilson, is more likely to be rewarded by profitable discovery.

I scarcely need do more than mention the great assistance which workers may obtain from the museum of this college. In the original Hunterian Collection there were 287 specimens of cancerous diseases. To these, 1200 have since been added. Microscopic specimens, showing the structure of various forms of these diseases in different organs and tissues, may also be studied in a collection of several hundred prepared by Mr. Eve, who has nearly finished a complete catalogue of the collection. The valuable collection of Hunterian drawings has been enriched, at the suggestion of Sir James Paget, by many illustrations of morbid anatomy. And, quite recently, Dr. Matthews Duncan has presented a large and beautifully executed collection of water-color drawings of cancerous and other diseases of the vulva. Some of them are on the table, and will, I hope, stimulate many to follow so good an example.

Although the hour is rapidly approaching its end, I must not pass over without remark recent discussions as to the supposed microbic origin of cancerous growths. Cases of acute cancerosis or miliary cancer, analogous to acute tuberculosis or miliary tubercle, have led to the search for a specific microbe, or bacillus. Scheurlen believes he has found one, but nearly all those who have examined his statements have been led rather to negative than to confirm his conclusions. Senger, indeed, has almost proved that Scheurlen's cancer bacillus is nothing more than a potato bacillus—one which grows readily on slices of potato, and is often accidentally found there. So far as inoculation experiments, or grafting of portions of cancerous growths upon sound parts of the body, have hitherto gone, they are certainly against the microbic doctrine. We can only admit that any disease is caused by a microbe when the micro-organism has been isolated, has been cultivated outside the human body, and then, when the cultured organism has been introduced, it has led to an identical form of disease or growth. Unless these three things are done we have no positive proof that a disease is due to specific germs.

Knowing how keenly such questions as these are now discussed, I was anxious to know if the great leader of German pathologists has yet arrived at any definite conclusion regarding them. So I wrote to Professor Virchow, and he replied on October 25 last, sending me a paper published in his Archives on the "Diagnosis and Prognosis of Carcinoma," and adding, "Since I wrote that paper last December, the only progress in the knowledge of Scheurlen's bacillus was its detection growing on potato sections without cancerous origin." Professor Virchow also refers me especially to a part of his paper which expresses his present belief that "the most scrutinizing investigations have not yet arrived at a convincing demonstration." But, with equal caution, he adds that the possibility of the existence of such a micro-organism cannot simply be denied; and that the discovery of a specific bacillus would be of the greatest importance in the diagnosis and prognosis of carcinoma, because, he says, "The attempt to explain all the stages of cancer proliferation with dissemination and metastasis by the dispersion of cancer cells is by no means so certainly supported by anatomical or experimental proof as to exclude any other mode of explanation. Nor, on the other hand, is the need for a cancer bacillus so great that without it we are deprived of the possibility of understanding the process. Animal or human cells, quite as well as bacteria, have the power of influencing metamorphosis, and of producing effective secreted matters of the most various kinds. Why, then, should such an influence be denied to cancer cells, which in many, and especially in the worst cases, are in such a marked degree endowed with the character of gland-cells?"

I would refer any who may wish to study this part of the subject to some extremely valuable papers by Mr. Ballance and Mr. Shattock published in the Pathological Transactions for this year and last year, and especially to their reports of cultivation experiments with malignant new growths made to the Collective Investigation Committee of the British Medical Association. Although in their attempts to propagate the disease by inoculation they have not yet succeeded, they still hold ("British Medical Journal," October 29, 1887) that "the parasitic theory in some form or other is the most probable of any of those yet advanced." What they now desire is that inoculated animals should be kept for the full term of their natural life under healthy sanitary conditions; as the life-history of the parasite may be a long one, and it may be a long time before the characteristic effects of inoculation could be expected.

The time at my disposal is so very short that I must at once pass on to the consideration of our duty as surgeons in treating sufferers from cancerous diseases, and I propose to ask you to reflect at your leisure upon certain questions about which the mind of the profession is still not definitely settled, rather than to accept any conclusions of mine.

The first of these questions is whether a cancerous growth alone, or the whole of the part or organ which it has invaded, should be removed; and I think the time has come to agree upon some general rule or principle of treatment. With regard to cancer of the breast, two very opposite opinions are held by men of high position as hospital surgeons. Mr. Nunn, after very large experience at the Middlesex Hospital, in his admirable treatise on " Cancer of the Breast," says .(p. 32): " When an operation has been decided upon, the removal of the entire mammary gland must be complete, any partial removal is not only useless but worse than useless; the occurrence of the slightest speck of cancer in a gland declares that the whole organ is more or less ready for special degeneration." Mr. Butlin, whose experience at St. Bartholomew's is also very large, and whose work on the operative surgery of malignant disease is rich in facts carefully tested and in conclusions drawn with remarkable judgment and freedom from prejudice, takes a very different position to that of Mr. Nunn. He says that in many cases the tumors are "at first of small size, limited to a part of the breast, often situated toward the margin of the gland " (p. 381); and he adds: " Just as good reason could, I am sure, be given for the removal of both breasts in every case of cancer of one of them, as for the removal of the entire mammary gland in every instance." Time prevents me from entering further upon this important practical question than to say that my own practice, and what I have actually seen of the practice of others during the past thirty years, would lead me to remove the entire breast in every case of cancer, except where the growths are small and close to the margin of the gland, or only affect outlying portions of the gland. And when such growths are found not in the gland, but in the axilla, I should strongly oppose removal of the breast, because I think such tumors may be neither of the breast itself nor of the axillary lymphatic glands, but of a certain class of sweat-glands which have been the subject of a paper by Dr. Creighton. I believe it is only necessary to direct more attention to this inquiry to lead to the recognition of a new and a large class of tumors of the axillary and pectoral regions.

The tumors to which I allude are found at the outer border of one or both breasts, and the surgeon is doubtful whether the breast itself is or is not involved in the new growth. When the growth is between the outer border of the mammary gland and the corresponding axilla, the fear is felt that the axillary glands are involved in the breast disease: and opinions are given that both the axillary tumors and the breast should be removed. Such a case came before me scarcely a month ago. On the 25th of last month, a married lady, who had never been pregnant, forty-six years of age, came to me from Wales, having had a strong opinion that her right breast should be removed without delay. I found both breasts larger and harder than usual, both nipples unusually large and prominent, but the only distinct tumor to be felt was between the upper and outer border of the right mamma and the axilla. Extending from this border, below and behind the pectoral muscle, was a round, movable, tender tumor about three inches in lateral and two in vertical measurement. It was in close connection with the mammary gland; but I thought I could separate one from the other. The patient felt sure that a blow from a tennis ball two years ago had been the cause of the swelling. I advised that neither of the breasts should be removed; but that the tumor or tumors, whatever they might be, should be removed without delay. Meeting Dr. Creighton later on the same day, I mentioned the case to him, and he at once suggested that the tumor might be neither of the breast nor of the axillary lymphatic glands, but of certain sweat-glands below the skin of the axilla which he had referred to in connection with tumors in a paper which was read at the Royal Medical and Chirurgical Society six years ago, and may be found in the sixty-fifth volume of the Transactions of the Society. In that paper he shows that the special layer of glandular substance more or less developed in the human axilla, corresponds to a conglobate form of gland not previously described, in one of the lowest mammalians, with an invest-ment of unstriped muscular fibres in parallel order around each crypt, so as to constitute a basement membrane upon which the epithelial cells are seated. These sweat-glands differ in important respects from the ordinary skin glands of man. They are not usually in the substance of the skin, but adhere to its under surface, lying between the skin and the axillary

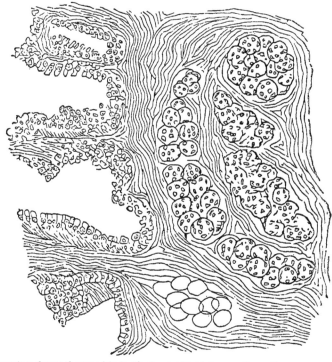

This drawing shows the two kinds of gland structure exactly as they are seen in one of Dr. Creighton's preparations. To the right is seen a portion of a mammary lobule in a rest-ing state; and, on the left, a scattered deposit of the so-called sweat-glands, with muscular basement membrane.

fascia, and sometimes extending to the lateral and anterior regions of the chest. They are variously developed in differ-ent individuals, and must be regarded as a sort of survival or rudimentary organ, and subject to all the risks of such sur-vivals or rudiments. Dr. Creighton says: " I have, in one in-stance, found perfect examples of them in intimate association with the breast structure."

I show you here the tumor which I removed entire on Octo-ber 30, as well as the fragments of another somewhat smaller

tumor, and the tissue I removed in dissecting away the invest-
ing membrane after the interior had been cleared out. Dr.
Creighton was present, and made a careful examination on
the same day of all that I removed. The smaller or pectoral
tumor was so closely connected with the breast that I removed
with it a small piece of the outer border of the gland, enough
to show that the breast itself was quite healthy. In order to
be sure of removing the whole of the tumors, I removed some
of the surrounding fat also, and Dr. Creighton reported to me
that he found "embedded" in the fat, round, reddish bodies,
about the size of a large pin-head. "One of these, easily extracted from the surrounding fat, proved to be a coil or cluster
of the tubular axillary glands of perfectly normal structure,
in which the characteristic palisade-like basement membrane
of unstriped muscular fibres, the mosaic of polyhedric epithelium resting on the latter, and the conglobate windings and
crypt-like recesses of the tubule were easily seen in a preparation of the fresh tissue. The capsule of the smaller and more
friable new growth adhered along the axillary side of the
piece of fat, the normal reddish cluster of glands lying in the
fat about an eighth of an inch deeper. This capsule was everywhere infiltrated with blood; its inner surface was not uniform,
but subdivided into a number of round areas or recesses of
unequal size, one or two of which were specially marked by
their black pigmentation. The examination of that capsular
tissue, and of the friable tumor tissue which was removed from
it by the finger during the operation, discovered satisfactory
evidence of the same glandular structure as in the small reddish body embedded in the adjoining fat—namely, unstriped
muscular fibres, spherical or polyhedric epithelium, with or
without brown or black pigment, and, in sections, traces of the
tubular glands themselves.

"The larger mass of tumor was situated deeper in the axilla, and was unconnected with the portion nearest to the
breast, except by loose tissue. It was extracted by the fingers
entire, an encapsuled lobulated oval body, about two and a
half inches in its long axis, and an inch and a quarter across
at its thicker end. The surface was everywhere dark red, giving it some resemblance to a small kidney. In its lobulation
it looked like a packet of lymphatic glands. On section it
proved to be a whitish medullary substance with a few small

areas of pigmentation, and with a general foliaceous or lobulated arrangement of the stroma. In microscopic preparations of the fresh tissue, unmistakable examples of unstriped muscular fibres were found, as well as the same polyhedric and spherical epithelium, with and without pigment, as in the more friable tumor nearer to the breast. In sections the epithelial cells were found collected in alveolar heaps, generally of great extent. The dark color of the capsule was from infiltration of blood."

The general structure of these tumors of the irregularly scattered sweat-glands, including their hæmorrhagic capsule, appears to be the same that has been described for the puzzling class of cases known as "alveolar sarcoma of the breast," or "duct-cancer of the breast." It is noteworthy that these cases have sometimes been found to start from the areola around the nipple, a region which is known to be provided with the same kind of tubular glands as are found in the axilla. When such growths ulcerate they resemble rodent ulcer. The so-called eczema of the nipple, which has been observed in such cases, would appear to be connected with the orifices of the gland, and, in its simpler forms, to be little more than the brownish secretion of the glands dried upon the skin. It seems probable that this case, and Dr. Creighton's observations upon it, will be the beginning of a new classification— or of the separation of such cases from the class of mammary tumors, and their reference to the irregular deposits of sweat-glands of the axilla, and to the glands of the areola.

I may add that a tube draining away from the axilla was kept in for three days, and after its removal union of the incision, about four inches long, was complete when the sutures were removed. The patient returned to Wales a few days after the operation. I have arranged for a report as to any recurrence hereafter, but venture upon a favorable prognosis.

Again, we may be consulted in cases where the period for early and hopeful operation has passed by, or where, months or years after operation, recurrence has taken place—it may be that recurring growths have also been removed, once or several times—and then comes a time when a patient, exhansted by loss of blood, or by profuse offensive discharge, approaches the end, and further operative treatment is abandoned. Are we to be content with relieving pain, prolonging sleep, and the use of deodorizing or disinfecting appliances, or can we do more? Can we encourage the forlorn hope of the patient that growth may still be stopped? that some benign alteration may take place in its structure—something like the "spontaneous involution" of Virchow—some retrograde fatty change in the cells or elementary components of the tumor, while extension or growth of new cancer cells is stopped? If this could be attained before other parts of the body were infected it would amount to curing cancer. From time to time such cases of cure are reported, but few, if any, stand the test of accurate investigation. Virchow, however, cautions us against too great scepticism in such therapeutical investigations, and says that the hopeless condition of the patient justifies the trial of remedies of whose mode of action we have no clear idea. Whether we can go still further, and secure for healthy tissues immunity against infection from an existing cancer—a resistance to invasion—remains a subject for future inquiry. All we can yet say is, that under certain conditions the nutrition of cancer cells may be so far arrested as to lead to their complete disintegration. This is often observed in small fragments, or within a limited circumference, and Nussbaum has recently succeeded in the attempt to effect such changes in larger growths by cutting off their supply of blood. He makes deep furrows with Paquelin's cautery through the integuments and subcutaneous fat quite down to the adjacent fascia or muscles, thus cuts off all peripheral supply of blood, and so lessens the abnormal vascularity of many malignant tumors. Soft fungoid masses which bleed readily soon become firm, and the whole tumor more solid, while the general health improves and life is prolonged. And we also hear from Munich of aims at a somewhat similar object by injecting solutions of ozone into the substance of cancerous growths and the tissues surrounding them. Not only is the proliferation of the epithelial cells said to be arrested, and the formation of cicatricial tissue obtained, but the surrounding textures are protected against invasion. So long as the disease is local it must be curable. As Virchow says in concluding his last paper, "If cancer in its beginning, and often very long afterward, is a local disease, it must be possible during this period locally to cure it."

When a superficial cancer on a limb has returned after destruction by cauterization or caustics, or after removal by the knife and grafting of healthy skin, and the lymphatic glands nearer the body remain free from infection, the propriety of amptating the limb must become the subject for consultation. It will sometimes be the painful duty of the surgeon to urge upon a reluctant patient to sacrifice a limb in the hope of saving life; and if this advice is followed before infection of the glands has taken place, the result has often proved the soundness of the advice; while too great delay, or want of earnestness in urging submission to so serious an alternative as the loss of a limb must always be, may lead to protracted suffering and inevitable death.

I have yet another subject for your consideration, one which the general public enters into with a good deal of warm feeling and an amount of ignorance which calls rather for instruction than blame. I mean the removal of cancerous growths by cauterization instead of by the knife. On this point let me read to you what our great master, John Hunter, said just a hundred years ago (Palmer's edition of his works, vol. i., page 625) as to cures for cancer:

"No cure has yet been found: for what I call a cure is an alteration of the disposition and the effect of that disposition, and not the destruction of the cancerous parts. But as we have no such medicine, we are often obliged to remove cancerous parts, which extirpation, however, will often cure as well as we could do by changing the disposition and action. Arsenic seems to have some power of this kind, and its effects might be increased, by being used internally and externally; but its use is very dangerous, and I am afraid insufficient for the disease. This is a remedy which enters into the empirical nostrums which are in vogue for curing cancer; and among which Plunkett's holds the highest rank. But this is no new discovery, for Senertus, who lived the Lord knows how long ago, mentions a Roderiguez and Flusius, who obtained considerable fame and fortune by such a composition. I was desired to meet Mr. Plunkett, to decide on the propriety of using his medicine in a particular case. I have no objection to meet anybody. It was the young one: the old one is dead, and might have died himself of a cancer for aught I know. I asked him what he intended to do with his medicine. He said, 'To cure the patient.' 'Let me know what you mean by that. Do you mean to alter the diseased state of the parts, or do

you mean by your medicine to remove the parts diseased?'
'I mean to destroy them,' he replied. 'Well, then, that is
nothing more than I or any other surgeon can do with less
pain to the patient.' Poor Woollett, the engraver, died under
one of these cancer-curers; he was under my care when this
person took him in hand. He had been a life-guardsman, I
think, and had got a never-failing receipt. I continued to call
on Woollett as a friend, and received great accounts of the
good effects, upon hearing which I said, if the man would give
me leave to watch regularly the appearance of the cancer and
see myself the good effects, and should be satisfied of its curing only that cancer (mind, not by destroying it), I would
exert all my power to make him the richest man in the kingdom. But he would have nothing to do with me, and tortured
poor Woollett for some time, till at last I heard the sound
testicle was gone, and at length he died."

How this story of John Hunter reminds us of much that
goes on every year in this great city! More than thirty years
ago, in 1857, I published a lecture on the cancer-curers of that
day—Pattison and Fell, Landolfi and the Black doctor, Bever-
edge and the Rev. Hugh Reed. I believe the exposure of Mr.
Reed's practice did much to prevent other cancer-curers from
doing much harm in London. But there are still irregular
practitioners heard of, who follow the line of Plunkett, Pattison, and Fell, who profess not only to destroy a cancerous
tumor, but also what they call its roots, and thus prevent a
return; or, as Fell professed, to destroy the "tendency existing in many cases in the constitution for the reproduction of
cancerous cells," and to "destroy the cancerous diathesis."
It is curious to compare this claim with John Hunter's remarks on the use of arsenic to "destroy the cancerous disposition," with Mr. Hutchinson's recent observations on "Arsenic-
Cancer," and with Dr. Creighton's views on arsenic among
other alterative or "habit-breaking" drugs, metals, or metal-
loid substances having elective affinities for particular tissues;
and this theory of cancer as an acquired habit of the tissues,
"a habit that might be broken if we only knew how." The
inhalation of oxygen and the use of oxygenated water as a
beverage have been supported upon somewhat similar grounds,
and did no harm beyond disappointing the patient. But as a
fashion its day was short. The use of methodical compression,

which often did good, has led to the more modern *massage,* which has already done much harm. On looking over my old lecture I find this sentence: " I should not be at all surprised to hear that the next great empiric who appears in London will profess to cure cancer by galvanism." I have been surprised that this advent has been so long delayed, although there have been proofs of late that female galvanic doctors are at work, and others calling themselves electro-homœopaths, doing some harm, but not deserving the title of great empirics. While writing this, I hear of certain cancer-curers whose head-quarters are at Brussels, but who have correspondents in London and Southampton, whose practice leads to results quite as bad as any of those of Pattison and Fell. I must not pursue this rather tempting subject further than to repeat my assertion that " we have no reason to fear a comparison between what we can do by fair and open means and what really can be done or ever has been done by any cancer-curer or any secret remedy."

More than ten years ago, in June 1878, lecturing in this theatre, I gave a short account of Freund's method of entirely removing a cancerous uterus through an incision in the abdominal wall, and referred to Blundell's four cases of removal through the vagina. I then said I thought it would be rarely that an entire uterus affected by cancer would be removed by laparotomy; and I need now only add that the results of the practice have been so disappointing that it may be said to be practically abandoned. I have only twice removed the entire uterus by laparotomy, and the specimens in both cases are on the table before you. One is of some historical interest as having been the first instance in his country of excision of the entire gravid uterus. The patient was six months pregnant and suffered from epithelioma of the cervix uteri. You see the entire uterus and the ovaries, just as they were removed, and the opening through which the fœtus was extracted. The patient recovered from the operation and was in fairly good health for several months; but the disease recurred in the left iliac fossa, and death took place thirteen months after operation. The other case was much more satisfactory. A patient at the full term of pregnancy had her pelvis so blocked up by a uterine tumor that delivery was impossible. You see the uterus which I removed with both ovaries, and the cavity from which a living child was extracted. Recovery was as rapid as after a natural labor, and I received a photograph of· mother and child a year after the operation, both being quite well. I need say no more of these cases, as they have both been published, except that they have proved that in case of need the entire uterus, containing a fœtus or a viable child, with considerable tumors, and with both ovaries, may be successfully removed through the abdominal wall.

Removal through the vagina is a much more successful operation. It did not attract serious attention in England until after a discussion at the Obstetrical Society in March, 1885, where it may be said to have been generally condemned. In the report of that discussion I find the following remarks of my own:—

"It is to be hoped that at least as good results may be obtained here as in Germany, and that condemnation of the principle of the operation will not be the verdict of the Obstetrical Society. Have we sufficient facts before us to justify such a verdict? Admitting that abdominal extirpations have resulted in a mortality of 72 per cent., and vaginal extirpations of 28 per cent., is it to be supposed that improved methods will not lead to diminishing mortality? Admitting that recurrence of the disease within a few months, or, at most, in from two to five years, has hitherto been the rule, may not a more accurate diagnosis, earlier operations, and improving methods lead to better results; not only to a lower death-rate, but to a retarded recurrence and sometimes to complete recovery?"

It will hardly be disputed now that the mode of operating has been improved and that mortality has diminished; and I think I cannot employ the few minutes still allotted to me better than in rapidly sketching what I believe to be the best mode of operating, and in bringing before you the results already attained by experienced operators.

But I must first say a few words comparing removal of the entire uterus with removal of the diseased part only, by the operations known as infra-vaginal and supra-vaginal amputations. The diagrams on the next page show what is meant by these alternative proceedings.

Of course it must be difficult to draw a very definite line, and say exactly where one or other of the two operations begins or ends, but these are near enough for all practical purposes, and if they are compared with this other diagram after Freund, showing what is done when the entire uterus is removed, both Fallopian tubes and both ovaries being left

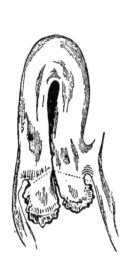
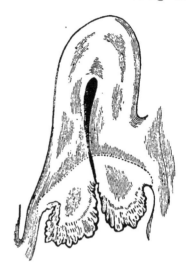

behind, a very good idea may be formed as to the comparative gravity of the different procedures.

In many cases of total extirpation it may be advisable to remove both Fallopian tubes as well as the uterus, and in

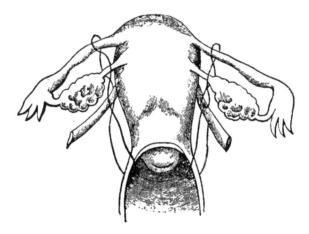

some cases one or both ovaries should also be removed. This will, I need hardly say, depend upon the healthy or diseased condition of the different parts.

I am sure we are not yet in a position to compare numerically the risks of partial or total excisions neither as regards the immediate danger of death from the operation nor as to the liability to recurrence at longer or shorter intervals. This must be done at some future time when we have a larger number of cases accurately observed and faithfully recorded. At present I can only offer a general statement that in my own practice, when the disease is strictly limited to the parts near the os, I prefer infra-vaginal amputation, and I do it by the galvanic cautery écraseur, using the wire at a low red heat, and tightening the loop very slowly. I have removed nearly the whole of the cervix in this way without losing one drop of blood. A white dry eschar is left, and cicatrization follows without fever or much pain. When disease has extended rather higher, amputation must be done with knife or scissors, but it is well to cauterize the raw or bleeding surfaces by copper or gas cautery or Paquelin's, to serve the double purpose of checking bleeding and destroying any infective cells that may possibly have invaded the tissues above the line of amputation.

Before passing on to the details of the operation of total excision, I must say a few words as to the use of caustics rather than the knife, scissors, or cautery. Potassa fusa has been largely used in this way, and I have heard of, but never seen, very good results following. And I have seen several cases treated by the late Dr. Wynn Williams with bromine. But not one ended satisfactorily, although temporary good was done. On the table is a very remarkable specimen of the entire uterus which sloughed away after the use of chloride of zinc. Dr. Marion Sims carefully scraped away with his curette all the diseased structure till he came upon hard uterine tissue. Then he applied persulphate of iron upon cotton wool, left this for twenty-four hours, removed the styptic plug, applied another plug of wool charged with a strong solution of chloride of zinc, and left this for four days. After removing this plug, antiseptic vaginal injections were used for several days, and then I found this mass quite loose in the vagina. It consists of the entire uterus, and when fresh it was quite evident that some of the peritoneal coat of the fundus came away with it. The patient suffered a great deal, and died about two months after the application of the caustic; sooner, I believe, than if she had been left alone.

After what I have said it cannot be surprising that in any case where cancerous disease has extended much higher than the os, and there is good reason to believe from the mobility of the organ that the surrounding tissues are still free from invasion, I advise total excision as the best practice. And increasing experience is materially simplifying the operation. I cannot pretend now to describe the different steps in detail, and I need only allude to the importance of preliminary disinfection of the vagina, removal of any dead or softening cauliflower excrescences, and shaving off all hair from pubes and vulva. This may be done the day before operation.

During the operation the patient is fixed in the lithotomy position by anklets and wristbands, or by a thigh crutch; and a douche and elastic tube are so arranged that a stream of warm, slightly-carbolized water may continually irrigate the vagina. The body is well covered, as well as the arms, legs, and feet, to prevent chilling. If the uterus is fairly mobile, no speculum is required, at most one or two retractors. Some operators draw down the uterus by a simple or double hook, or by hooked forceps; but if the cervix is firm, any friable part having been cleared away, the safest plan is to pass a strong wire quite through the cervix. This is safe, and not so likely to be cut as silk. Supposing that any intention of turning the fundus either forward or backward is, as it ought to be, abandoned, the cervix is pulled by the wire toward the vulvar orifice, the labia held aside, and the sides of the vagina separated if necessary. The operation is completed by different stages.

1. Division and loosening, and pushing up to the extent of half to three quarters of an inch, of the vaginal mucous membrane behind and in front of the cervix.

2. Pushing upward or separation of the bladder and ureters from the neck and anterior surface of the body of the uterus.

3. Opening Douglas's pouch, and introduction of a sponge to keep up the small intestines.

4. Securing the uterine arteries on both sides by ligature or by pressure forceps.

5. Division of the broad ligaments and other attachments, and removal of the uterus.

6. Cleansing vagina, removal of sponges, arranging ligature threads or forceps, and loose plugging with iodoform gauze.

It is unnecessary to such an audience as this to enter into further detail; but I will refer briefly to two matters of great importance—the safety of the bladder and ureters, and the substitution of forcipressure for the ligature.

Sometimes the separation of the bladder from the uterus is quite easy, sometimes very difficult, and I am sure great care is always required to avoid the ureters. In several re-

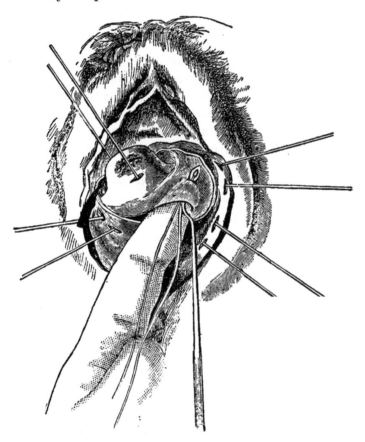

corded cases one, and in more than one case both ureters have been tied or divided. I need hardly remind you that one mode of death in uterine cancer is uræmic coma, caused by closing up of one of both ureters. And I show you here the parts removed after the death of a patient from uræmic coma. She was operated upon by a very experienced American surgeon for vesico-vaginal fistula, yet one ureter was included in the sutures which closed the fistula, and the other was left opening into the vagina behind the united edges of the fistula. In some recorded cases the bladder has been wounded, and in others the catheter or sound passed through the urethra, and used as a guide to the separating finger or to pull the bladder forward, has been seen through the thin muscular coat and mucous membrane of the bladder.

In one of these drawings the mode of passing one of the ligatures used to secure the uterine arteries is shown—a threaded blunt needle is guided by one finger passed into Douglas's pouch. One or more may afterward be passed in

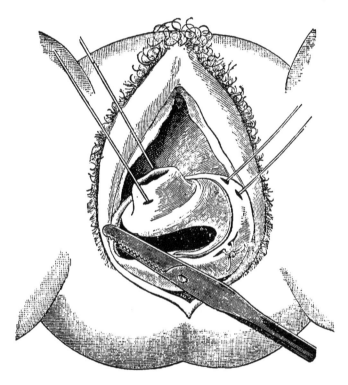

the same way to secure the broad ligament on either side, or the same object may be gained by the use of pressure-forceps, as shown in the next drawing. These are not removed, but are left on for twenty-four, thirty-six, or forty-eight hours until all danger of bleeding has ceased. Leopold and some German operators prefer the ligature. Péan, Richelot, and other Frenchmen trust to the forceps. I believe I was the first to suggest their use, and one of our Fellows, Mr. Jennings, the first in this country to carry out the suggestion with success. Some warm controversy has arisen in Paris lately on this matter, and Dr. Pozzi, in a small work on vaginal hysterectomy for cancer just published puts the historical question as follows. After quoting what I wrote in 1882 ("Ovarian and Uterine Tumors," p. 526) recommending the "securing any bleeding vessel as it is divided by pressure-forceps, not using any ligatures, but leaving the forceps hanging out of the vagina for two or three days until all danger of hemorrhage has ceased," Dr. Pozzi refers to Mr. Jennings's successful case in October, 1885, before M. Richelot's first case in April, 1886, but after M. Péan's first in June, 1885, which was not published until April, 1886, and concludes that, although M. Richelot has "vulgarized" forcipressure in this operation, Mr. Jennings's case had been published nine months before M. Richelot made his communication to the Academy of Medicine.

But it matters very little who first proposed or first practiced a particular method. The chief thing is to decide whether it should be followed or not, and my own belief is that it must be left to the choice of the surgeon in each case. He should be prepared to secure bleeding vessels by ligature or the forceps, as he finds he can do it more easily. Forceps with a variety of curves may prove more convenient than the straight instrument shown in the drawing. It may be that ligatures will do all that is required, and the best way of applying them that of Leopold, as shown in the drawing, each ligature passing twice through the peritoneum of Douglas's pouch and the vagina, and being tied so as to lie parallel to the line of incision—not simply bringing serous and mucous edges together, but compressing in separate portions the whole of the vaginal wall. I think the quickest way to do this would be to have a long ligature threaded at each end on a small needle, which would be passed by a needle-holder from the serous outward through the mucous membrane.

When these ligatures are tied they form a chain of compression all round the edges, and may be used afterward by loosely tying some or all of the long ends together to close the opening from the vagina into the peritoneal cavity as far as may be desirable. By crossing their handles pressure forceps would have the same effect. My own feeling would be rather to trust as a rule to forceps, and only exceptionally to ligatures. Forcipressure is simpler, more secure, takes much less time, and saves much suffering to the patient when sutures are removed. When an operator, who has prepared himself for the operation by sufficient practice on the dead body, trusts to forcipressure and has arranged everything before he begins, I feel sure that fifteen or twenty minutes would give ample time to complete the operation if the ovaries are not disturbed. If healthy, I think they had better be left alone, and so may the Fallopian tubes. But if the disease has extended high up the uterine cavity it would be safe to remove the tubes. And this would add very little to the duration of the operation.

I shall not attempt to give the results of this operation statistically; but it is important that we should know what a few of the most experienced operators have been able to accomplish. Professor Olshausen, of Berlin, formerly of Halle, who has had probably a larger experience of this operation than any other surgeon, informs me that the following table represents the whole of his experience of total extirpation of the uterus *per vaginam* for cancer:—

Years.		Operations.	Deaths.
1881–82	(beside five incomplete operations, which all recovered)	22	8
From Jan 1, 1883, to April 30, 1887	(no complete operation) . . .	31	5
	Total operations in Halle . .	53	13
From May 1, 1887, to Nov. 5, 1888	Total operations in Berlin . .	99	13
	Total	152	26

The Professor adds: "I very seldom perform supra-vaginal amputation, and only when the carcinoma is limited to the *portio vaginalis*. Of my cases done in 1881–82, I have one who has remained free from recurrence for seven years, two others have been free for five and a half years, and one for five years. Professor Leopold wrote to me on the 11th of this month, stating that up to that date he had performed total extirpation of the uterus by the vagina in eighty-three cases with only five deaths, a mortality of six per cent. Péan, writing on the 13th, says that from 1882 to the end of 1887 he had done twenty-two operations, fifteen successful, and with seven deaths; but that this year he has had sixteen cases, all successful and no deaths. Martin, of Berlin, who had previously published sixty-six cases where cancer led to the operation, with eleven deaths, or sixteen per cent. mortality, writes on the 16th of this month: "Since the Washington Congress in 1887, I have performed the vaginal total operation in twenty-two instances." (He does not say in how many for cancer.) "All recovered but one, who died of hæmorrhage. Of supravaginal amputation I performed altogether six, with one death." It would be easy to collect a very large number of cases: such as Schroeder, fifty-nine, with five per cent. mortality; Fritsch sixty, also seven per cent. But these do not bring us later than 1866, and they all tell the same story of greater success following larger experience.

As to the comparative mortality of infra- and supra-vaginal amputation and total excision, the results vary so much in successive years and in the practice of different operators that I have been unable to collect materials for a trustworthy contrast either as to the immediate fatality or as to the frequency of recurrence of disease. But it certainly appears that recurrence is earlier after partial than after complete operations. In some series the remarkable fact comes out that supravaginal amputation stands the test of recurrence better than complete excision. This would be inexplicable if it were not for the probability that the disease had been generally much further advanced in the cases where total excision was performed than in the others.

Our American brethren have been before us in adopting the operation of total excision of the uterus, and, as elsewhere, their results have improved with time and experience.

The cases hitherto performed in this country have not been enough to serve for any comparison of results with those abroad, but they all teach the lesson that if the operation is to be successful it must be done early, before surrounding structures are involved in the disease. In addition to the case of Mr. Jennings, of which I have spoken, Dr. Purcell has had five successful cases; Dr. Sinclair, of Manchester, four; Mr. Reeves, Dr. W. Duncan, and Dr. Keith, one each; and I dare say other cases might be found by searching the medical journals of the last three or four years.

There are other parts of this subject on which I should like to say much more. I have alluded to Mr. Haviland's work on the geographical distribution of cancer, and now I can only point to these two of his maps which show how in certain districts of this country the mortality from cancer is high, and from phthisis low, and the exact reverse in other districts. I wished to allude to cancerous disease of the ovary, and to say how difficult it is to decide whether an ovarian tumor is innocent or malignant, even after it has been removed and carefully examined. Now I can do no more than support the rule to operate early as the best way to avoid recurrence. I wished also to remind you how the mortality after amputation of the breast, and after removal of other parts affected by cancerous disease, has been so much lessened by modern sanitary science that all the old arguments against operating at all in cases of cancer require revision. I wished to say something about inadequate operations, and about operations which are unnecessarily severe—and much more than I did say against operating in hopeless cases, and in studying how to "soothe where we cannot save." Of cases which especially interest us, where cancer has affected the lips or tongue, the œsophagus, the larynx, the pylorus, the spleen or kidneys, the intestines, the bladder, and the female genital organs, I have not time to say another word. And now, in conclusion, I will only venture to express the belief that if some who have heard or who may read this lecture are convinced that cancer is increasing will try to find out the cause of the increase, and why cancerous diseases are so prevalent and so fatal; if they will also try to learn how to prevent or to cure them, no one can forecast the result. No one could have imagined that a forgotten book of Marco Polo would rouse the spirit of research in Columbus and lead to the discovery of a new continent, and no one can foretell what the work of one man may accomplish. It may be trifling, but—

> Think nought a trifle, though it small appear;
> Small sands the mountain, moments make the year,
> And trifles Life.

Each one may bring an offering, however small, to the altar of one of the temples of Æsculapius—or, if his own search for knowledge fail, he may assist in preventing the failure of others, and in guiding them along the path to full success. And, year after year, the Morton Lecture may exert some influence for good upon all mankind in all coming generations.

CARDIAC DYSPNŒA

AND CARDIAC ASTHMA

BY

PROF. DR. S. von BASCH

CARDIAC DYSPNŒA AND CARDIAC ASTHMA.

I. Pathology of Cardiac Dyspnœa.

WE apply the term dyspnœal to those forms of respiration in which increased exertion of the respiratory muscles is observed. This exertion occurs either in the work of the inspiratory muscles alone, or in that of the expiratory muscles, or in that of both. We distinguish, accordingly, inspiratory, expiratory, and general dyspnœa.

The impeded respiration may be present, although it is not brought to the notice of consciousness in an increased degree. This is called objective dyspnœa. But the impeded respiration may reach consciousness as a feeling of want of breath and in this event the dyspnœa is also subjective.

Dyspnœa may be the result of various causes.

If we disregard those causes which depend on diseases of the nervous respiratory centre and consider only those which affect the respiratory mechanism itself, we must first speak of the dyspnœa resulting from obstruction to the current of air in the upper air passages, the larynx and trachea, and in the larger and smaller bronchi.

Dyspnœa may also result from diminution of the respiratory surface proper of the lung, *i.e.*, the complex of the alveoli, by fluid due to inflammation, chronic and acute, or to catarrhal diseases of the mucous membrane. Distention of the lung may also be obstructed by compression from the outside, such as pleuritic exudation, the atmospheric pressure (pneumothorax) and tumors. Finally the diminished elasticity of the pulmonary alveoli, which renders impossible the return of the pulmonary volume to the normal, may also lead to dyspnœa.

All these forms do not belong directly within the field of our inquiry. We will here discuss only that variety of dyspnœa in which the changes of the pulmonary mechanism, which have just been mentioned, are not the real causes, but the increased distention of the pulmonary vessels with blood is the immediate cause of the dyspnœa.

As it is the changed mechanism of the heart which leads to the increased fulness of the vessels, it seems to me to be expedient, and also justifiable from a clinical standpoint, to apply the term "cardiac dyspnœa" to this variety. That form of asthma which depends upon changes in the cardiac mechanism and which will be fully discussed later, is called cardiac asthma.

Much is said concerning cardiac dyspnœa, although not under this term, in the oldest and recent writings on diseases of the heart. It is unanimously described as the first and most important symptom of a developing disease of the heart, and there is hardly a disease, whether it affects the heart muscle itself, the pericardium, endocardium or valvular lesions associated therewith, in which it is not fully referred to as an accompanying symptom.

As regards the clinical interpretation of this symptom, we have hitherto been satisfied with the conception that the distention of the pulmonary vessels is a symptom of stasis. The relation of this stasis to the dyspnœa was sought in the slowing of the current of blood in the lungs, which interferes with the interchange of gases, in the diminution of space in the alveoli by the capillaries which are filled with blood and project into the alveolar space, and finally in the accumulation of secretion in the alveoli and bronchi, which was attributed to the stasis and known as stasis-catarrh.

A clinical picture that is not satisfied with describing a symptom, with pointing to the anatomical disturbances in the organs that are involved, but also attempts to afford an explanation of the biological processes that take part, may not be content with the general explanations and conceptions hitherto offered. It must embrace all the considerations that may serve to clear up and widen our views concerning the biological processes. It is in this way alone that the diagnosis *i.e.*, our recognition of a pathological condition, can correspond to the present status of medical science, which is built up by clinical, anatomical, and physiological experiences.

The clinical consideration of cardiac dyspnœa must start with physiological dyspnœa, *i.e.*, with the causes which produce dyspnœa in healthy individuals when they perform an unusual amount of work.

There is one physiological fact from which the discussion must start, and this fact, which I and others have determined by sphygmomanometric measurement, is the following: "the arterial pressure is increased by bodily exertion."

This increase occurs, as we may assume, in the following way:

The muscular work increases the amount of carbonic acid in the blood. Although the interchange of gases in the lungs is not changed by the muscular action, the blood thus acquires a dyspnœic character, therefore stimulates the vaso-motor centres, produces contractions in the vessels and thus leads to increase of the blood-pressure. As the respiratory centre also reacts, in the well-known manner, to the irritation of the dyspnœic blood, the respiratory movements become deeper and more rapid. This might secure a regulation, inasmuch as the deep and accelerated respiration might be able to remove the excess of carbonic acid produced by the muscular action, and to supply the greater amount of oxygen required.

But this regulation, as every one can experience by experimenting on himself, is insufficient, and the dyspnœa increases with continued forced movements, despite the respiratory strain.

Hitherto I had been unable to answer the question, why the dyspnœa continues, otherwise than with the assumption that the left heart exceeds the limits of its power of accommodation with the increasing resistance in the vessels, and that, when this happens, the left ventricle no longer empties its contents completely. Hence, the left auricle is more than usually filled with blood and, as a result, the blood is dammed back in the lungs.

But this view was opposed by the results of measurement of the blood-pressure. When I produced very marked dyspnœa in myself by rapidly climbing a mountain and made the measurements in the midst of the most marked dyspnœa, the pressure of the blood was found to be very high, and by no means falling. This did not favor the opinion that my heart was unable to overcome the resistance of the vessels, since, if this were true, the blood-pressure would fall at the height of the dyspnœa.

My opinions, which accorded with the current conceptions of the relations of dyspnœa to blood stasis in the lungs, must therefore present an hiatus, and I was forced to the suspicion that the high blood-pressure *per se* and not the stasis in the lungs—which can only develop in a higher grade when the blood-pressure sinks—was a cause of the dyspnœa.

This suspicion was correct. Reflection, supported by undeniable facts, shows that the respiratory capacity of the lungs must suffer when, together with the increased pressure in the arteries, the pressure in the pulmonary artery also rises, as does actually happen.

In a recent article "Ueber eine Funktion des Capillardruckes in den Lungen" (Wiener med. Blätter, 1887, No. 15) I have shown that the walls of the pulmonary alveoli become more rigid when the capillaries imbedded in them are filled under high pressure, and that the respiratory capacity of the lungs is diminished by increase of this pressure.

In order to make this understood, I must here enter more fully into the subject.

Sufficient air ventilation in the lungs can be conceived only under the assumption that the volume of the alveoli is considerably increased during inspiration and correspondingly diminished during expiration. The bronchi and infundibula have little to do with the ventilation because they form cavities surrounded by comparatively rigid walls. As the result of this their lumen does not change materially, entirely apart from the fact that their structure is incapable of respiration. The greater the excursion of an alveolus and hence of the lung as a whole, the greater is the amount of moved air that is employed in ventilation of the blood. Whatever impedes these excursions must, as is easily seen, impair the respiratory power of the lungs.

Upon what does the amount of these excursions depend?

If we assume that the lungs are emptied of blood—this does not happen during life—then the diminution in the size of the alveolus would be the result of the elastic and tonic properties of the tissue elements in the alveolar walls; the enlargement of the alveolus would result from the traction of the inspiratory muscles, which oppose the elastic forces.

What happens when the pulmonary capillaries that surround the alveoli are filled with blood? Is the condition of the alveoli the same as when the lung is destitute of blood? By no means. In a measure, the filled capillaries cause erection of the alveolus; it becomes larger, its lumen increases, and its walls grow more rigid. The forces which are to dilate it during inspiration must therefore become greater and it cannot return to the same volume during expiration as a bloodless alveolus. The great difference between a lung whose vessels are empty and one whose vessels are filled, is shown by a simple experiment that I have recently performed.

The lungs with the heart are removed from the thorax of an animal, and the pulmonary artery together with the left auricle, into which the pulmonary veins empty, are provided with canulæ. At the same time fluid is forced into the lungs through the pulmonary artery from a vessel under pressure and the trachea is connected with a bellows that is regularly opened and closed. It will then be found that, when the bellows is set in motion, the lungs are distended to a certain extent with each descent of the bellows. If fluid is now allowed to enter the pulmonary vessels, it is first noticed that the lungs grow larger and, if the bellows are again used, the lungs will be distended less than before. If the trachea has been connected with a water manometer before this second distention and before the injection, we can also convince ourselves that the enlargement of the lungs after the injection does not depend upon the passage of fluid into the alveoli, inasmuch as the fluid sinks in the manometer, *i.e.*, the lungs exercise suction while enlarging, and this suction can only depend upon the fact that the space inclosed by the alveolar walls has become larger.

The fact that increased distention of the vessels causes erection of the tissues within which they are inclosed and makes them more rigid, is well known. Whoever has made or seen an artificial injection, could convince himself of this. But no one has thought heretofore of erection of the alveoli and its relations to respiration. It happened to me that I did not understand experiments (of which I will speak later) which were made under my observation and direction and which, as I now see, clearly showed that the filling of the pulmonary capillaries under increased pressure interferes with the distention of the lungs. I was still imbued with the old idea that only the diminution in the size of the alveoli or their filling with fluid can interfere with the entrance of air into the lungs.

The alveolus or lung, whose vessels are filled with blood, acts accordingly in an entirely different manner from the lung which is empty of blood. It was not necessary for me to demonstrate this. The proof was found in the figures obtained from measurements made on the lungs of dead bodies by Donders and on the lung of the living animal by Jakobson and Adamkiewicz. These figures differ from one another in a notable degree.

The lung of the dead body exercises upon the closed thorax a traction which corresponds to the pressure of seven and one-half millimetres mercury. In the living animal this traction is much less, viz., three to five millimetres mercury. This shows clearly that the living lung, filled with blood, returns during expiration to a much less volume than the lung which is empty of blood.

The difference between the experiments of Donders and those of Jakobson and Adamkiewicz have not been interpreted hitherto in this manner. We have satisfied ourselves with the notion that the elasticity of the lungs in man is different from that in animals. It is unnecessary to enter into details in order to show that this notion is not correct.

The lung, whose capillaries are filled with blood, will therefore be larger in rest during expiration than the lung which is empty of blood or the lung of the dead body. As the elasticity[1] of the alveolar wall increases with the distention of the capillaries and consequently its distensibility diminishes, the forces which distend a lung filled with blood must be greater,

---

[1] According to the doctrines of physics, a body is so much more elastic the greater the force or weight required to distend it to a certain extent. A rod of steel of a certain diameter is, in this sense, more elastic than a rubber cylinder of the same diameter. The distensibility of a body is, therefore, not in a direct but in an inverse proportion to its elasticity. The easily distended rubber cylinder is, in a physical sense, less elastic than the, with difficulty distensible, steel rod. As a matter of course, the rigidity of a body increases with its elasticity.

because the rigidity of the alveolar wall has increased with its elasticity.

Under normal circulatory conditions, in which the pulmonary capillaries are only exposed to a moderate pressure (concerning whose amount we possess no positive knowledge) the inspiratory muscular power is entirely sufficient, we must assume, to produce the distention necessary to sufficient ventilation.

It is clear that this force is required in an increased measure, when the pressure in the pulmonary artery increases and with it the pressure in the pulmonary capillaries. Such an increase may occur in two ways. The pressure in the pulmonary artery may increase with increasing pressure in the aorta or with diminishing pressure in that vessel.

In the consideration of physiological dyspnœa, the discussion of which we will now resume, a part is played only by the first factor, *i.e.*, the increase of the capillary pressure in the lungs, as the result of increased pressure in the arteries. How shall we conceive the mode of development of physiological dyspnœa? The starting point is the increase of arterial blood-pressure, as the result of narrowing of the vessels. If we enter more closely into the circulatory processes which attend the increase of arterial pressure—not on the basis of speculative consideration, as unfortunately happens very often, but on that of positive experimental experience—it will be found that this increase is almost always followed by a back action which causes an increase of pressure in the left auricle, in the pulmonary artery, and also in the veins. This is clearly evident from experiments in which the changes mentioned are observed after manipulations that increase the arterial pressure. I may refer to experiments that have been made in the Physiological Institute of Leipzig, by Waller under the direction of Ludwig, then by Openchowsky under Stricker's supervision. Lichtheim and I have made numerous experiments in this direction. Increase of pressure by irritation of the cervical cord distends the left auricle with blood to such an extent that its movements cease. As the result of dyspnœal irritation of the vessels in suffocation, the pressure of the pulmonary artery increases with that of the aorta, and, as I know, the pulmonary pressure also increases when the increased aortic pressure has been produced in a reflex manner. It has

also been known to me for three years, from experiments made
by Dr. Schweinburg under my direction, that the increased
aortic pressure resulting from strychnine is followed by a very
considerable increase of the venous pressure. In the increase
of pressure in the aorta which is caused chiefly by narrowing
of the small arteries, the two halves of the heart, the tract of
the lesser circulation situated between them, and the vessels
of the greater circulation are more filled with blood than the
small arteries and capillaries of those tracts that are affected
by spasm. In this changed condition of the pressure and distribution of the blood, the lungs, as is readily seen, are most
affected because every increase of pressure in their vessels
means an increase in rigidity of the alveoli, and thus an im-
pairment of the respiratory functions. The development of
dyspnœa in increase of arterial pressure is now explained very
easily. If dyspnœa does not occur on forced muscular movement, the reason may be seen in the following considerations.
In the first place, it is possible that the rigid alveoli are sufficiently distended by greater traction of the respiratory
muscles during inspiration, and that, as this corresponds to
the greater amount of blood which flows through the lungs in
a more rapid current, a greater movement of air in the lungs
takes place by means of which the poverty of oxygen and
the increase of carbonic acid in the lungs are prevented. This
at least explains the fact that forced muscular movements
which increase the blood-pressure do not produce the feeling
of dyspnœa. Furthermore, as is self-evident, the muscular
movement will not produce dyspnœa when it does not give
rise to increased pressure in the arteries, or when such increase
is very slight. Numerous experiments in this direction are
wanting, but we will hardly go astray in concluding from the
experiments hitherto made that habit here plays a great part;
at least the well-known fact that even skilled mountain climb-
ers, after they have rested for a long time, must, so to speak,
train for long trips by smaller ones, is explained easily by the
assumption that the irritability of the vaso-motor centres to
the stimulus produced by muscular movement is diminished
after prolonged action. In this sense I would interpret the
statement of Oertel who by means of my sphygmomanometer
demonstrated upon his patient, Dr. N., a greater increase of
pressure after the first mountain climb than after subsequent

ones. In the same sense I would also interpret the experiments made by Marey upon horses. He found that the blood-pressure not alone does not rise during work, but even sinks. He is inclined to generalize this result, and extend it to men, but in my opinion without justification. The horse is a beast of burden, and is by no means to be compared with man. When the latter is unused to work, he is especially apt to suffer from palpitation of the heart, and from shortness of breath on increased effort. Yet we should examine whether working-people do not act like the horse so far as regards their blood-pressure. It is shown, however, by the reports of autopsies upon racing horses and hunted deer, in whom colossal hypertrophy of the heart was found, that even in these animals a great increase of blood-pressure must occur as the result of excessive strain.

Dyspnœa after bodily exertion is a cardiac dyspnœa. So long as its development can be attributed to unusually great stimuli, it is to be regarded as physiological. The term pathological cardiac dyspnœa may only be used when slight causes suffice to produce it. If we hold fast to the view that the swelling of the lungs and their rigidity constitute the primary factor, the relative insufficiency of the muscular respiratory apparatus, the secondary factor, which produce cardiac dyspnœa when acting together, we can readily understand that in the different cases a greater etiological importance attaches sometimes to one, sometimes to the other factor. We have learned that excessive bodily movement, which under certain circumstances increases the blood-pressure in a high degree, is the cause of physiological cardiac dyspnœa. We must now concern ourselves with those causes which also give rise to increased blood-pressure, and come into play in pathological cardiac dyspnœa. Bodily movement, but not excessive, is among the first of these causes. We must consider not alone the character of each movement, but also the work produced. A strong bodily movement in a muscular, but lean individual by no means indicates the same effect as a comparatively slight effort in individuals whose muscles are weak, but who possess a large deposit of adipose. This difference will be especially felt in lifting the entire weight of the body, for example, in ascending a mountain. If a lean individual gets out of breath in walking up a flight of stairs, we must infer a greater disturbance of the circulatory apparatus than when this happens under similar circumstances in a very stout individual. The increased work of the heart in such cases is often associated with the feeling of palpitation of the heart, but palpitation is by no means a constant symptom in dyspnœa resulting from movement. Increase of blood-pressure also occurs in changes of the position of the body. In standing the blood-pressure is less than in the recumbent position, as various experiments have proven. The increase of blood-pressure on lying down may therefore be a cause of the development of cardiac dyspnœa, and this corresponds perfectly to clinical experience. The dyspnœa which develops on lying down is usually, though not always, associated with the feeling of palpitation of the heart. Mental excitement, cutaneous reflexes as the result of thermal actions, such as baths, douches, etc., may also cause increase of the blood-pressure This increase is often preceded by palpitation. Dyspnœa very often occurs with the palpitation, and is probably connected with the increase of blood-pressure. Palpitation and dyspnœa may also result from toxic action, such as that of coffee, tobacco, etc. We must now ask how it happens that slight increase of pressure in the arteries is followed by a comparatively great increase in the pulmonary and the capillaries of the alveoli, and thus impairs the respiratory capacity of the lungs to a considerable extent. As I have become convinced from protracted observation, sphygmomanometric measurements are of special value in the consideration of the condition of the patient. If these measurements show normal pressure, and if examination also shows that the frequency of the pulse is normal, and that the size, beat and sounds of the heart present no abnormal condition, and if we also find—assuming that the lungs themselves furnish no cause for respiratory disturbance—that the tendency to dyspnœa is nevertheless present, this can only reside in two causes. In the first place, there may be abnormal irritability of the vascular system which causes very great increase of blood-pressure after slight causes. If this is not the case, as must appear from the examination, the cause can reside only in an insufficiency of the heart, which may occur despite apparently normal findings. In absolute or relative rest of the body, this insufficiency is not manifested. Its effect is shown at once when the heart is required to perform increased labor.

If for any reason there is a slight increase of resistance in the arteries, and therefore a slight increase of blood-pressure in the pulmonary, then, if the left heart is able to do the increased work, *i.e.*, to empty itself completely—assuming that the regulating activity of the respiratory muscles is entirely intact—there is no occasion for the occurrence of dyspnœa. But such an occasion arises at once, if the pressure in the pulmonary artery or capillaries increases to a comparatively greater extent than that in the arteries. This must occur at once when the left ventricle becomes insufficient, *i.e.*, when it evacuates its contents incompletely. If this happens, then the pressure in the left auricle, whose contents cannot be evacuated completely into the left ventricle, must increase, inasmuch as the ventricle is fuller than normal at the close of systole and the beginning diastole. As a result, the pressure in the pulmonary artery and capillaries must increase. I need no longer enforce the fact that this increase entails greater swelling of the lungs and greater rigidity.

Measurements may also show a sub-normal pressure in the arteries. In such cases we must first consider whether the low blood-pressure is associated with normal or abnormal distribution of the blood. If the distribution is normal, *i.e.*, if the low pressure depends upon the slight resistance in the arterial tracts, and the cause for the slowed current of blood must be sought outside of the heart, then the same considerations hold good as before with regard to the development of dyspnœa. From the height of the blood-pressure alone we cannot infer directly that the action of the heart is insufficient, inasmuch as many cases are observed in which there is no disposition to dyspnœa, despite low blood-pressure, *i.e.*, in which a heart that normally does little work suffices entirely for increased work. If dyspnœa occurs in such cases in which the blood-pressure is lowered, then we have to deal either with abnormal irritability of the vascular system, or relative insufficiency of the left ventricle. It is different when the low pressure develops in combination with a changed distribution of the blood, *i.e.*, when the arteries are less distended because the veins and the lesser circulation contain comparatively more blood. Whether this is true must be determined from the condition of the veins of the neck, and of the other veins, especially in the lower extremities, in which varices or even

slight œdematous swellings occur, but particularly from the
condition of the heart itself. Intensification of the second pulmonary sound, a. difference in the intensity of the sounds of
the left and right heart, enlargement of the heart toward the
sternum also favor the view that the low arterial pressure depends upon weakness of the heart.   One of the most important
data consists in the very great predisposition to shortness of
breath.   This is very easily explained.   With the changed distribution of the blood the pressure in the pulmonary artery
and capillaries increases.   The lungs of individuals with weak
hearts must therefore be larger and more rigid from the start,
and the limit at which the rigidity reaches a stage when the
work of the respiratory muscles is no longer sufficient will
very soon be passed.   This no longer requires, as in the former
cases, increased stimuli or increased blood-pressure in the
arteries, because, inasmuch as the heart is insufficient from
the start, the slightest increased work of the left ventricle
must be remarkably noticeable in the pulmonary circulation.
In addition, there is the important fact that the transition
from a high grade of pulmonary rigidity or elasticity to a still
higher one takes place, not in arithmetical, but in geometri-
cal progression, *i.e.*, that the distensibility of the lungs diminishes in a still more marked degree in the higher grades of
distention with blood.   The same remarks hold good with regard to those cases in which the changed distribution of the
blood is produced by valvular lesions in which a lower blood-
pressure is found.   It is evident that a valvular lesion, so far
as regards its general effect upon the distribution of blood, is
equivalent to insufficiency of the heart because in certain
of these cases the left ventricle at systole throws into the
arteries only a part of the blood which has collected in the left
auricle during its diastole.

In excessive arterial pressure, predisposition to dyspnœa
will always be considerable because the high arterial pressure
is accompanied by high pressure in the pulmonary artery, and
therefore by increased rigidity of the lungs.   This corresponds
to the clinical experience that a very great tendency to cardiac dyspnœa is shown by individuals in whom high arterial
tension is observed, whether as the result of arterio-sclerosis
or of chronic nephritis or retraction of the kidneys, or of both
together.   Here, as in all cases in which the pulmonary ves-

sels are filled under higher pressure, the volume of the lungs will be comparatively greater on account of the condition of swelling of the organ.

The predisposition to dyspnœa increases still more when the pressure in the pulmonary artery and left auricle is greatly increased. This may happen when, as the result of very great frictional resistance in the arteries in severe arterio-sclerosis, the current of blood in the arteries and capillaries is very slow, and hence the veins and lesser circulation are filled under relatively higher pressure. Such a condition would be shown by pronounced swelling and pulsation of the cervical veins.

Finally, relative increase of the pressure in the pulmonary artery may also result from insufficiency of the heart muscle. In this event, increased fulness and pulsation of the veins of the neck will again be one of the characteristic symptoms. Hypertrophy of the heart, even when it has reached a high degree, does not exclude the possibility of such insufficiency, because a strong predisposition to dyspnœa and pronounced venous pulsation are observed particularly in cases of hypertrophy of the left heart.

In addition to the condition of the lungs which develops as the result of the circulatory disturbance just mentioned, we must also consider the condition of the respiratory mechanism situated outside of the lungs. Its unimpaired functions may in some degree compensate for the obstruction to respiration due to the lungs themselves. Pari passu with diminished distensibility of the lung, the inspiratory muscles may vigorously dilate the space within which the lungs are inclosed to a greater extent; furthermore, the expiratory muscles which, as a rule, are at rest during normal respiration because expiration is effected solely by the elastic force of the thorax and lungs, now also come into action and aid in diminishing the size of the lungs.

Wherever the conditions for the production of this compensation are absent, cardiac dyspnœa must develop more easily under otherwise similar circulatory conditions.

In the first place, respiration may be relatively insufficient on account of weakness of the respiratory muscles. This may occur in emaciated individuals and those reduced by severe disease. In general lipomatosis, it may also happen that the diaphragm and intercostal muscles undergo fatty degenera-

7—4

tion, like the other muscles of the body. To Germain Sée belongs the credit of having called attention to this important point. In pseudo-hypertrophy of the muscles, it is also possible that the degeneration may produce respiratory insufficiency. The activity of the respiratory muscles may also be interfered with by obstacles to the distention of the thorax. This is the case in horizontal decubitus, in which the thorax rests upon a firm base, and the excursions of the ribs are impeded by friction. The obstacles to the distention of the thorax may also result from the elevation of the diaphragm, as the result of abnormal fulness of the abdominal cavity (distention of the intestines by gas and fluid accumulation in the abdomen, tumors, etc.). Finally the excursions of the thorax may be hindered by deformity resulting from curvature of the spine, rachitic changes in the ribs, adhesions after exudations, etc. I disregard entirely those processes which involve the lungs themselves, because they are no longer instances of pure cardiac dyspnœa.

II. Pathology of Cardiac Asthma.

The asthmatic attack is distinguished from dyspnœa by its sudden, but, above all, by its spontaneous occurrence. In cardiac dyspnœa the external causes are known in every case while the cardiac asthmatic attack develops apparently without any visible cause. I say apparently, because such causes surely exist, as is shown by reflection and observation.

In what do the causes of this sudden occurrence of cardiac asthma consist?

We must first distinguish between the attacks that appear during the day and those that appear at night. The nocturnal attacks may again be differentiated. The attack may occur as soon as the patient lies down, *i.e.*, before he falls asleep or shortly after falling asleep, *i.e.*, in the first slumber, before sleep is profound, or finally in the middle of the night during deep sleep.

We will start with the last case and discuss the causes of an attack of cardiac asthma occurring in deep sleep; we will then consider the processes present at this time in the circulation, *i.e.*, in the heart, vessels, and lungs.

Traube properly called attention to the fact that the superficial character of respiration during sleep is the chief cause of the development of the asthmatic attack. In addition we must take into consideration the fact discovered by Burdon-Sanderson that the rima glottidis is narrowed during sleep on account of relaxation of the laryngeal muscles.

How do these two factors aid in the production of the seizure ?

When respiration is superficial and the rima glottidis narrow, the respiratory process, *i.e.*, the interchange of gases in the blood, will be less active than in the waking condition. It is sufficient, as a rule, because the need of oyxgen is much less in complete rest of the body, and the excretion of carbonic acid is not so abundant. But the degree of fulness of the pulmonary vessels must play a part during sleep as well as in the waking condition. If the pulmonary vessels are relatively less full during sleep, the superficial respiration will more readily suffice for the respiratory needs than when the pulmonary vessels are fuller.

Our knowledge of the condition of the blood-pressure during sleep is very slight. From experiments which I made some years ago with the pletismographic method, I learned that the volume of the arm diminished during sleep. I attributed this to lowering of the blood-pressure. My experiments were made during the day upon patients in a surgical ward.

On the other hand, Mosso has observed increased volume of the arm during nocturnal sleep. So far as I can judge of the changes in volume, this would testify in favor of an increase of the blood-pressure. Unfortunately I have had no opportunity of making such observations with the sphygmomanometer.

If we take into consideration that the blood-pressure is greater, in general, in the recumbent position, it cannot be denied that an increase of pressure may occur during sleep. If this happened, the superficial respiration, which occurs as the result of sleep, would become relatively insufficient, *i.e.*, it would not suffice for the increased rigidity of the lungs and would lead to dyspnœa. It is also conceivable that the respiration is more than usually superficial in certain cases and that this would lead to dyspnœa without the aid of increased pressure.

The dyspnœa which has thus developed, whether in one

way or the other, would give rise to increase of the blood pressure. In the first event, the already higher pressure will become still higher, and in the second event, the normal blood-pressure will be increased.

As I conceive, these are the prodromes which may be followed by the asthmatic attack.

In this preliminary stage, which may develop without reaching the patient's consciousness, the processes are identical with those during cardiac dyspnœa. In both cases the increased blood-pressure in the arteries causes rigidity and swelling of the lungs, but in the former the increased pressure occurs during bodily rest, in the latter it is produced during bodily movement.

It is easily understood that the unfavorable effect of the swelling of the lungs upon respiration is much more marked during sleep than during the waking condition. In sleep, the insufficiency of the respiratory mechanism is a normal phenomenon, and on account of this insufficiency the compensation on the part of the respiratory mechanism remains absent in part. I say in part, because the possibility is not excluded that dyspnœal intensified respiratory movements may occur during sleep. In the waking condition, however, the compensation will always be more complete because the freer position of the thorax favors its distention and because the automatic impulses, which start from the medulla oblongata, are reinforced by voluntary impulses which, as we may assume, increase the work of the respiratory muscles.

Traube had called special attention to the importance of the will in respiration. He properly maintains that orthopnœa, *i.e.*, the condition in which the patient voluntarily attempts to increase the effect of respiration by a more favorable position of the body, constitutes a much more favorable condition of respiration than that in which the already somnolent patient is no longer able to sit up and does not feel the shortness of breath, although this is very intense, as shown by the cyanosis. What Traube says of somnolence is also true, in a measure, of sleep.

These considerations also favor the assumption that dyspnœa and its results (increase of blood-pressure and pulmonary rigidity) can develop much more suddenly during sleep than in the waking condition, and easily explain the fact that the patients are not roused from sleep until the dyspnœa has reached a very high grade.

So long as the sudden dyspnœa continues under high blood-pressure, so long, in my opinion, it should be regarded as the prodromal stage of asthma. The term asthma should only be applied to that condition in which the heart has changed its condition of equilibrium and in which the distention of the pulmonary vessels no longer depends upon increased pressure in the arteries, but is associated with considerable diminution of pressure. Here again Traube first recognized the truth and made the very apt remark that, in the development of the asthmatic attack, we have to deal with a labile condition of the heart.

In what manner can the heart fall from its condition of equilibrium?

We will discuss this question upon the basis of our physiological knowledge and the results furnished by clinical examination.

The experimental material at our command is tolerably assured, but the clinical material has been insufficiently utilized in this direction, because the conceptions which should guide clinical observation have been wanting hitherto. For this reason I speak only of an attempt to explain the production of cardiac asthma. An explanation, which is also satisfactory from a clinical standpoint, can only be given when it turns out that the results of clinical observation and post-mortem examination are in thorough harmony with those of experiments.

As the latter show, the change in the condition of equilibrium of the heart may occur in two forms, as paresis or paralysis of the heart, and as spasm of the heart.

The former can be studied experimentally in suffocation, the latter in muscarin poisoning. Both forms furnish the basis for the notions that guide us in comprehending the processes that occur in cardiac asthma.

If artificial respiration is interrupted in a curarized animal whose respiration is maintained artificially by blowing air into the lungs, the animal is left to the action of the blood of suffocation, and we can examine the processes in the right and left halves of the circulation, as Openchowsky showed and as I have often seen and demonstrated. With the increase of pressure in the aorta during suffocation—a long known fact—the pressure in the pulmonary artery (which had fallen temporarily at the beginning of suffocation) also rises. In the further course of the suffocation, at a time when the pressure in the artery is falling to a marked extent, the pressure in the pulmonary artery again increases, to an even greater extent than at the beginning.

Observation of the exposed heart, in addition to measurement of the pressure in the aorta, pulmonary artery and the auricles, sufficiently explains what takes place in the heart and circulation during suffocation. At first, when the pressure in the aorta and pulmonary artery is high, the heart appears uniformly distended in both halves. Both ventricles pulsate vigorously and sufficiently, but soon the left ventricle and auricle (the latter to a less extent) begin to dilate, while the right ventricle, on the other hand, grows smaller. The contractions of the left ventricle diminish somewhat in vigor with its dilatation, and at this time it is found that the pressure in the carotids is diminishing. The contractions of the right ventricle have apparently lost none of their vigor at this time. It is only at a very late period, when only slight contractions, which run across the surface like waves, are visible upon the surface of the left ventricle, that the contractions of the right ventricle also grow more feeble.

This condition of the heart is the result of paresis, due, in its turn, to the blood of suffocation. In such a case we cannot speak of paralysis because, on resuming artificial respiration, the heart soon returns to the shape and mode of action which it had shortly after suffocation. The heart can only be regarded as paralyzed in such experiments when it can no longer be restored by artificial respiration, *i.e.*, by supplying oxygenated blood. In a paralyzed heart, the wave-like contractions of the left heart and the feeble contractions of the right heart grow constantly smaller and finally cease, despite artificial respiration.

Why does the left ventricle alone dilate after the injurious action of the toxic dyspnœal blood? Undoubtedly because the two halves of the heart do not react in the same way to the toxic blood.

As a result of the weaker action of the left ventricle, not alone does it no longer throw its contents completely into the arteries, but a part remains in the ventricle at the close of systole. Hence the diastolic distention of the left ventricle gradually increases and, at the same time, the right ventricle, which receives its blood indirectly from the arteries, is filled less and less. The action of the right ventricle long suffices to expel the constantly diminishing amount of blood which it receives from the left heart and hence the left heart continues to be filled by the right heart.

On account of this increase of pressure in the left auricle, —which results from two factors, the uninterrupted supply from the lungs and the obstructed passage into the left ventriele, which is becoming more and more filled and can no longer empty itself on account of the weakness of its muscular tissue—the pressure in the pulmonary vein increases at a time when that in the arteries is diminishing considerably.

As the pressure in the pulmonary vein and left auricle increases with the increasing paresis of the heart, the pressure in the pulmonary capillaries must also be very high and hence a high degree of swelling and rigidity of the lungs may develop.[1]

Like the cessation of artificial respiration in the curarized animal, so the dyspnœa of the prodromal stage of asthma in man may change the blood in such a way that it produces paresis, and the heart may thus fall into the condition which we have just described.

---

[1] I have spoken of unlike reaction of both halves of the heart to the blood of suffocation. This unlikeness may be only apparent. It is possible that the left ventricle becomes larger because its power diminishes under distention of its walls. This distention would result from the resistance which the dyspnœally contracted vessels offer to the evacuation of the left ventricle. This resistance is present at a time when the arterial pressure is diminishing on account of the paresis of the heart, and when the paresis itself creates new conditions which also lead to increased filling of the left ventricle. The primary dilatation of the right ventricle at the beginning of suffocation is in great part the result of its increased fulness, and may disappear when the latter diminishes. This would explain the apparently dissimilar heart's action and the unequal size of both ventricles. On the other hand, it must be remembered that the left ventricle, as a rule, contains no dyspnœal blood, while this always forms the contents of the right ventricle. Upon this fact may also depend the greater sensibility of the left ventricle to dyspnœal blood.

The second form of disturbed equilibrium of the heart (spasm) is explained by the study of the processes observed in the heart and lungs of mammals after the introduction of muscarin. These experiments have been made by Dr. Grossmann in my laboratory and will be described exhaustively in the twelfth volume of the "Zeitschrift für Klinische Medicin." I will here refer only to what is absolutely indispensable in order to comprehend the subject.

If a solution of muscarin (one-half per cent) is injected into a curarized animal, whose respiration is maintained artificially, it will be found that the pressure in the arteries sinks but, at the same time, the pressure in both auricles and in the pulmonary artery increases. The increase of pressure in the left auricle is much greater than that occurring in Openchowsky's above-mentioned experiment. As the pressure phenomena are essentially the same as those observed in paresis of the heart from suffocation, it might be expected that muscarin paralyzes the heart. This is not so. The condition of the heart after the administration of muscarin is entirely different from that observed in an animal during suffocation.

When the exposed heart of an animal poisoned by muscarin is watched, it is found that the right ventricle, not the left, undergoes dilatation. The left ventricle appears small and contracted, and only the right heart and the two auricles, particularly the left, are distended with blood. The heart is in a spastic, not in a paretic condition. This spastic condition is more marked in the left ventricle than the right because the muscular tissue of the former is much more strongly developed than that of the latter. The muscular spasm diminishes the lumen of the left ventricle; hence during diastole, which is incomplete, the left ventricle cannot receive all the blood which flows from the distended left auricle and, although its systolic power is unchanged, it cannot fill the arteries sufficiently and produce high tension.

The right heart, as shown by its dilatation and the high pressure in the right auricle, still receives an abundant supply of blood and throws it into the lungs as shown by its vigorous contractions and the high pressure in the pulmonary artery. In the pulmonary vessels and capillaries, the blood is under very high pressure because its escape into the distended left auricle is interfered with. The pressure in the pulmonary capillaries attains such a height that transudation of fluid into the alveoli (œdema of the lungs) may result.

I cannot enter here into the proofs that the condition of the heart and the circulatory disturbances after the administration of muscarin really depend upon cardiac spasm, and must refer to Dr. Grossmann's treatise. We must emphasize the fact that the changes in the condition of the lungs in spasm of the heart are more profound than in paresis of the organ. This is evident indirectly from the condition of the blood-pressure in the lesser circulation. It can also be observed directly that the degree of pulmonary rigidity is much greater than that occurring as the result of suffocation and consequent paresis of the heart. The lungs of an animal poisoned with muscarin become so rigid that the air introduced is hardly able to distend them. But if the lung of an animal is tested, during suffocation, as regards distensibility (as I have seen in an experiment made by Schweinburg), it is found to suffer much less than in an animal poisoned with muscarin; in other words, the changes in volume of a lung filled with blood as the result of paresis of the heart differ to a less degree from the normal. This is in entire accord with the hydrodynamic conditions found on experiment; these show that, after paresis of the heart, the pulmonary capillaries are filled under less pressure than they are after spasm of the heart.

The difference between the two conditions as regards the distribution of the blood may be summed up as follows. In the paralytic condition of the heart, the blood in the greater circulation which has been thrown out of circulation is found in part in the lungs, in greater part in the left heart; in spasm of the heart, this blood is found in part in the right heart, in greater part in the lungs.

Of these two forms under which, as experiments show, the heart may change its condition of equilibrium, it may be assumed with certainty that the former possesses actual clinical significance. This view is favored by the fact that the dyspnœa produced by asthma has the same injurious action as suffocation has in experiments. The diminished respiratory capacity of the lungs is equivalent, under certain circumstances, to the cessation of artificial respiration.

Autopsical examinations also show, as I have learned from

authoritative sources (**Kundrat, Ed. v. Hoffmann**) that the left ventricle is found distended much more often than the right.

We must also ask whether the theory of cardiac spasm has any clinical justification. In other words, may the results of the experiments on animals be transferred to man and may it be assumed that there are forms of asthma which are attended with the development of spasm of the heart?

This was justifiable as regards paresis of the heart because we were warranted in inferring the same causes from the same effects—from the blood of suffocation as a cause, to paresis of the heart as an effect. Whether the blood of suffocation cannot act upon the heart in two ways, causing paralysis at one time and spasm at another, cannot be answered at present by experiment, and it must therefore be left in doubt whether dyspnœa as such may give rise to spasm of the heart.

But if we disregard cardiac spasm as the immediate cause of that condition in which the equilibrium of the heart is changed in such a way that the right and not the left ventricle undergoes dilatation, and if we look for another explanation of such a condition, we will easily find it if we assume that paresis of the heart may occur without dilatation of the left ventricle. The same cause, *i.e.*, dyspnœa, would then produce the same effects, viz., paresis of the heart. But this, according to our assumption, would vary in different cases. In one, which has been proven by experiment, the left ventricle would relax and dilate with the diminution in its contractile power, in the second supposed case its contractile power alone would diminish, but it would lose the power of dilatation; a sort of retraction might occur, independent of spasm. If this power of dilatation is lost, then the shape assumed by the heart must resemble that produced by spasm of the heart, *i.e.*, the right ventricle and left auricle must dilate (cardiac retraction is a phenomenon well known to experimenters and often seen in the frog. My assumption thus seems to be favored by the analogy).

The view that there may be a form of cardiac paresis whose results are analogous to those of cardiac spasm, does not disprove the opinion that spasm of the heart may also occur.

For the reasons just mentioned, the assumption of a cardiac spasm cannot be brought directly into association with dyspnœa, but with other causes which may give rise to a change in the condition of the heart. We must first think of causes of nervous origin.

It seems to me important, in this connection, to mention that angina pectoris, a disease attributed generally to a nervous origin, is regarded by many as a spasm of the heart. Heberden originally assumed a cardiac spasm in angina pectoris, and Dusch has adopted this theory. v. Bamberger also speaks of hyperkinesis of the heart in angina pectoris.

As I will show in detail in a paper on angina pectoris, those cases in which dyspnœal or asthmatic symptoms do not occur during the attack or are hardly noticeable, cannot be due to the same condition of the heart or lungs as in asthma. It is very possible, however, that in those cases of angina in which cardiac asthma plays a principal part, the latter may be due to spasm of the heart, like the pulmonary rigidity in muscarin poisoning. It is also possible that asthmatic attacks in which reflex irritation from the stomach, intestines, etc., is the primary or exciting factor, are the result of spasm of the heart. (The view that cardiac spasm is associated with nervous influences, is made very probable by experiments. The spasmodic condition of the heart in muscarin poisoning may be relieved, as Grossmann's experiments show, by irritation of the accelerator nerve. This favors the notion that muscarin produces the nervous spasm through the medium of nervous influences.)

To sum up in a few words, cardiac dyspnœa may place the heart in a paretic condition and thus produce cardiac asthma; furthermore, a primary spasm of the heart may develop and give rise to asthma. The first form must be called paralytic asthma, the second spasmodic asthma.

The assumption that the heart may pass into a condition like that described as spasm is also supported, so far as my knowledge goes, by post-mortem findings. After sudden death it is found not infrequently that the right heart, not the left heart, is enlarged considerably in its dimensions. As a matter of course, such findings do not teach us whether the left heart was undilated because it was attacked by spasm during life or because its muscular tissue was in a condition of retraction after paresis which did not permit dilatation of the left ventricle. At all events, according to these post-mortem appearances, spasm or retraction of the heart may be included among the possible conditions.

From the views here developed, it is self-evident that the condition of fulness of the heart, especially the left ventricle, plays a great part in the development of cardiac asthma. In a heart, whose left ventricle is very full and normally expels its blood under great resistance, the limits at which the heart can still respond to the increased demands will soon be reached as the result of further increase of the resistance. Paresis as well as spasm or retraction would here have a greater effect, because it would transfer a large amount of blood from the left into the right circulation. This agrees with clinical experience in so far as cardiac asthma occurs with special frequency under high arterial pressure, *i.e.*, in arterio-sclerosis and those valvular lesions which result from arterio-sclerosis such as aortic insufficiency and stenosis.

In addition to the high intercardial pressure, whose increase is apt to induce sudden over-distention of the heart and may lead temporarily to a condition like paralysis, it is to be remembered that, in arterio-sclerosis, the sclerotic process in the vessels, especially when it attacks the nutrient vessels of the heart, is apt to give rise to nutritive disturbances and pathological tissue changes in the heart and thus diminish its power of resistance.

In fact cardiac asthma, as Leyden has recently shown, is a very frequent symptom in sclerosis of the coronary arteries. In my opinion, however, cardiac asthma has nothing to do with sudden occlusion of the coronary artery. This leads to sudden paralysis, followed by death if permanent, by syncope if temporary, but in no event does dyspnœa or asthma follow sudden general cessation of the action of the heart.

In my remarks I have referred to those asthmatic attacks which appear during sound sleep. Asthma may also occur during the first sleep, and its causes are probably the same as in the former event. The stage of latency, however, is much shorter. Latency may be entirely wanting in those cases in which the asthma occurs during the day.

The exciting causes of diurnal asthma, as opposed to the nocturnal form, includes changed position of the body (recumbent position), bodily strain, mental and sexual excitement. I have seen cases in practice in which cardiac asthma occurred for the first time immediately after coitus. Further causal factors are distention of the stomach and intestines, and toxic influences. The latter include, in the first rank, those resulting from uræmia. It is also said that nicotine poisoning may give rise to cardiac asthma. I have seen no cases of this kind, although a number of instances have come under my observation in which nicotine poisoning produced cardiac symptoms (arhythmia, palpitation), and this cause undoubtedly takes part not infrequently in the production of angina pectoris. In severe cases of angina pectoris attended with cardiac asthma, when due to nicotine poisoning, the nicotine may be the indirect cause of the asthma. Chloral may also produce an attack of cardiac asthma, as I once observed.

The period of latency, *i.e.*, the development of the asthma, which attains its greatest intensity under falling blood-pressure, *i.e.*, under disturbance of the equilibrium of the heart's action, is not wanting here, but develops with the perfect consciousness of the patient. The course of the phenomena is probably the same as in nocturnal asthma, *i.e.*, the attack begins with high blood-pressure and consequent swelling of the lungs; it may remain at this stage or pass into a second stage characterized by low blood-pressure as the result of paresis, spasm, or retraction of the heart.

During the attack, the lungs may exhibit only swelling and rigidity or, as in muscarin poisoning, more or less extensive œdema may set in. Experiments lead us to infer that œdema of the lungs will develop in those cases in which the paresis of the heart occurs in that form which is analogous to spasm, *i.e.*, in the form of retraction. As is shown by the muscarin experiment, the conditions which give rise to œdema of the lungs, *i.e.*, the coincident increase of pressure in the pulmonary artery and left auricle, develop to the high degree which leads to œdema only when spasm of the heart occurs. In the cardiac spasm following the administration of muscarin, œdema of the lungs occurs; in suffocation paralysis of the heart, the lungs become swollen and rigid, but not œdematous. (The Cohnheim-Welch theory of pulmonary œdema cannot be maintained in its full sense. Œdema of the lungs cannot occur in early paralysis of the left ventricle, provided that the paralysis is complete and has led to dilatation of the left ventricle.)

III. Symptoms of Cardiac Dyspnœa.

THE main symptom is the feeling of want of air, which is present in greater or less severity. In the latter event, the patients are not thoroughly conscious of their condition. In describing their condition, they mention everything but the difficult breathing, and their attention is only called to it by direct questions.

As a rule, complaints concerning respiratory disturbances are heard only in more advanced cases, particularly when the want of breath is felt not alone after bodily strain—in this event it is not regarded by the patient as abnormal—but also when it appears to develop spontaneously. This happens generally after eating, especially after a hearty meal, when the difficulty of inspiring sufficient air is experienced during the ordinary, moderate movements. Patients who suffer from constipation state that walking is much more difficult on days when the bowels are not evacuated than on those in which a passage has been secured. Complaints concerning dyspnœa are also made when it attacks the patients after excitement, and they sometimes tell us that temporary annoying shortness of breath becomes noticeable after sexual excitement and coitus.

Respiratory disturbances appear very often in individuals in whom a rapid accumulation of fat, especially on the abdomen, has developed. I attach special importance to the latter circumstance, for in my experience, which has been very large in this direction, it is by no means true that individuals, who take on fat over the entire body, begin to suffer at once from shortness of breath.

Obesity may exist for years, it may even develop in individuals who are by no means sedentary in their habits and in whom, accordingly, external causes for the development of dyspnœa are not wanting (as in ardent hunters, workmen) without the occurrence of shortness of breath as a striking symptom. It is often not until the lapse of years that the obese individual complains of short breath, often at a time when the weight of the body is decreasing.

The manner in which the want of breath is perceived differs in different individuals. They sometimes complain of deficiency of air, hunger for air, sometimes that breathing is difficult. In the former event the respiratory activity does not appear to be obstructed, but the activity is ineffective and unsatisfactory, and is felt as such. In the second case the insufficiency of respiration, if I may so express myself, is felt directly. The patient says "breathing becomes difficult." In the first case, the patient feels as if he were performing a labor of Sisyphus; in the second case, he experiences the labored character of the increased work of the respiratory muscles. The feeling of want of breath is associated not infrequently with a feeling of oppression, constriction or pressure, but this does not always happen.

Palpitation of the heart is one of the associated symptoms of dyspnœa, but is by no means constant. There may even be very severe dyspnœa without a trace of palpitation. Others are observed in which a very slight degree of dyspnœa is accompanied by palpitation. When the latter symptom is present, it does not always begin with the dyspnœa. Sometimes the palpitation begins much earlier than the dypsnœa. At other times both appear at the same time, and finally the palpitation may not begin until long after the dyspnœa has developed. When the palpitation occurs with or during the dyspnœa, it must be assumed that both symptoms are related and they are to be regarded as the effect of the same cause, viz., the increased pressure in the arteries or pulmonary artery. I base this opinion upon the fact, repeatedly observed by me, that the blood-pressure increases during the palpitation, sometimes to a very considerable extent (thirty to fifty millimetres). When the dyspnœa does not appear until the palpitation has lasted a long time or is subsiding, we must be cautious in forming an opinion with regard to the respiratory condition. A year ago I had under observation a girl who suffered from palpitation of the heart and also complained of dyspnœa. Careful examination showed that this was not true dyspnœa. After the palpitation had lasted some time, the girl ceased to respire more deeply, indeed the respiration stopped entirely for a short time. This was not dyspnœa but apnœa, *i.e.*, a condition of absence of the desire for air. It resulted from the acceleration which the current of blood probably experienced during the palpitation and which caused over-ventilation of the blood in the lungs. The interpretation of this case depends upon an experiment made by Sigmund Mayer. If the peripheral extremity of one pneumogastric is irritated in an animal breathing voluntarily, dyspnœa first develops during the slowing of the pulse. After cessation of the irritation, when the frequency of the pulse becomes very great, the normal respiration first begins, but is soon interrupted by a prolonged apnœic interval. Sigmund Mayer properly attributes the dyspnœa to the slowness of the pulse, and regards the apnœa as a result of the accelerated current of blood with increased frequency of the pulse. I have observed a somewhat similar condition on irritating the accelerator nerve in an experiment, temporary cessation of respiration occurring during the irritation. In like manner, acceleration of the pulse in man, whether manifested by palpitation or not, might produce apnœa. This subject requires further clinical observation.

Patients who are attacked by dyspnœa on bodily movement attempt to escape it by remaining at rest, and this proves successful in all cases in which the bodily movement was the sole cause of the dyspnœa. Those who become dyspnœic in the horizontal position raise themselves in bed, and the erect position often suffices to relieve the dyspnæa. If the dyspnœa continues when the patient sits up and this position only affords relative relief, the condition is called orthopnœa.

Sitting up affords relief because the flow of blood from the large veins to the right heart is somewhat impeded, and the distention of the right heart cannot occur to the same extent as in the recumbent position. In addition, respiration is more free and unimpeded while sitting up, and the auxiliary efforts of the scaleni and sternomastoids can be brought into play by bracing the arms. This is impossible in dorsal decubitus. Finally, the diaphragm descends to a greater extent in the sitting posture, because the liver, stomach, and intestines sink from their own weight.

A strong desire to pass urine sometimes appears during dyspnœa.

IV. Symptoms of Cardiac Asthma.

Here the dyspnœa is very great; as a rule there is orthopnœa. The feeling of oppression is very distressing, the patients complain of a feeling of constriction of the chest and a heavy weight, with great anxiety, often intensified to a sensation of impending death. Cold sweat appears upon the forehead and body. As a rule, consciousness is entirely intact, but syncope sometimes occurs.

As in dyspnœa, palpitation of the heart accompanies the attack, but, as a rule, is felt only at the beginning. During the course of the attack, especially at its height, the palpitation falls into the background when compared with the other turbulent symptoms. The dyspnœa may be so severe as to make speech impossible. The patients become speechless but not aphasic. They fear to speak because inspiration is thus prolonged artificially and the active participation of the abdominal muscles is interfered with.

Involuntary micturition and even defecation sometimes occur during the attack.

The chief difference between dyspnœa and asthma consists in the conduct of the patients at the beginning and end of the attack. They attempt to escape dyspnœa by rest, but very often struggle against the asthmatic attack by movement. They jump out of bed, rush to the open window, walk up and down the room until they grow warm and perspiration breaks out. In very severe cases, however, in which the patients fall into a condition of great weakness, they must remain in the sitting position.

After an asthmatic attack the patient feels very exhausted and this may even persist until the following day. After dyspnœa he recovers in a little while.

V. Diagnosis of Cardiac Dyspnœa.

The first question concerns the diagnosis in the narrower sense, *i.e.*, whether the cause which lies at the bottom of the dyspnœa is essentially cardiac in character or whether the cardiac factor at least plays the principal part.

In order to answer this question, in general, we must examine for changes in the heart with the aid of physical methods. When valvular lesions are present, this examination will furnish a definite result, when they are not present, we must first direct our attention to changes in the size of the heart. These changes may be manifold in character.

Both sides of the heart may be enlarged; the enlargement may affect chiefly the right or left ventricle; or the auricles, particularly the left one, may undergo enlargement.

7—5

Such findings are very important in the diagnosis of cardiac dyspnœa, but to make it complete we must also ascertain the pressure in the arteries. A single measurement does not suffice to clear up the case. We must note whether, during bodily and mental rest, *i.e.*, at a time when the patient is not excited, the arterial pressure is decidedly lower than during moderate bodily movement or mental excitement; whether a change in the position of the body—passing from the erect position into horizontal decubitus—is followed by considerable increase in the blood-pressure. Such measurements also inform us concerning the degree of stability of the circulation, and we will learn whether the tendency to dyspnœa in the individual case coincides with such stability or its absence.

It is certainly of great value to combine measurement of the blood-pressure with the mapping out of the boundaries of the heart, as Scholl has done, because there is no doubt that the volume of the heart is as little constant as the blood-pressure. Scholl merits special praise for having shown the changeability of the size of the heart in a definite manner. This is not new to those who have had the opportunity of observing the exposed heart in living animals. On compression of the abdominal aorta the heart looks entirely different from what it does after compression of the vena cava. Irritation of the spinal cord and strychnine poisoning change the size of the heart materially; a heart that beats slowly looks different from one beating rapidly. If a patent example of the changeability in the shape of the heart is desired, let the experiment be made of bringing the organ under the influence of irritation of the pneumogastric and then under that of irritation of the accelerator; or watch the suffocation experiment, in which the heart is gradually paralyzed under the influence of the toxic action of the dyspnœic blood. The most surprising changes are exhibited when a heart poisoned with muscarin is again restored by atropine.

The changeability of the volume of the heart is not unknown to clinicians, but hitherto their attention has only been called to colossal enlargements of the heart or auricles, which appeared temporarily and then disappeared. Such cases have been described by Stokes and Traube, and Heiller described a case a few years ago. The latter constitute clinical rarities, and are not often seen in cardiac dyspnœa.

Although I am a firm believer in the variability of the size of the heart, I doubt the possibility of demonstrating this changeability upon the non-exposed heart with the aid of percussion in a positive manner.

This doubt is not based on a belief in the unreliability of the method of percussion or the skill of the observer, but upon the relations between the size of the lungs and the pressure in the pulmonary capillaries. If we assume that the pressure in the aorta is increased, two sets of changes in volume may occur, as is evident from our previous remarks. The increase of pressure may be associated with enlargement of both halves of the heart; this will happen when a normally acting heart is more filled than usual. In this event the heart and lungs become larger, and as the edges of the enlarged lung push across the heart, it may readily happen that the cardiac enlargement is not recognized. It may also happen that the heart grows smaller under increased pressure, and this will take place when the organ acted abnormally from the beginning, *i.e.*, exhibited a sort of insufficiency. When an insufficient heart begins to functionate normally, its volume grows smaller while the pressure in the arteries increases; in such cases only the arterial pressure rises, while the pulmonary pressure, which was relatively increased during the insufficiency of the heart, falls in comparison. Prior to such an event percussion might have appeared to show that the really enlarged heart was not enlarged, because the organ was covered to a greater extent by the enlarged lungs. Later, when the heart and lungs have become smaller, percussion is very apt to lead to the conclusion that the really small heart has become larger; the area of dulness is very apt to be increased by the retraction of the lungs.

Similar statements hold good with regard to the results of percussion of the heart, when the pressure in the arteries is low or falling.

Fall of the blood-pressure under normal conditions signifies diminution in the size of the heart and also of the lungs. Percussion may then mistake a larger heart for the really smaller one. Vice versa, when the arterial pressure falls as the result of cardiac insufficiency (and therefore the pulmonary pressure increases), the heart and lungs grow larger, while the heart may appear smaller on percussion.

I have made only one experiment similar to those of Scholl, and am therefore unable to state the amount of error that may arise from these relations. That such errors do exist may not alone be inferred *a priori* from theoretical considerations, but can be clearly proven clinically, as I showed recently in a case at the Policlinic under the control of my assistant, Dr. Schweinburg. In this case—arterio-sclerosis with cardiac dyspnœa—I mapped out the boundaries of the heart while the patient was breathing quietly. I then allowed him to walk rapidly about the room until dyspnœa developed, which occurred very soon in this case. Percussion during the dyspnœa showed that the heart had become decidedly smaller. Prior to the dyspnœa the dulness extended on the left side to more than one centimetre beyond the mammary line, on the right side to the middle of the sternum. During the dyspnœa the dulness began about two centimetres within the mammary line and extended only to the edge of the sternum. This diminution was certainly only apparent and depended upon the fact that the enlarged lung covered the heart more than before. It is more probable that the heart was enlarged, inasmuch as the arterial pressure had increased about twenty millimetres during the dyspnœa.

Future clinical examinations must take these errors into consideration. It is possible that in the measurement of relative cardiac dulness by percussion (in which we attempt to ascertain the absolute size of the heart) these errors do not impair the examination to such an extent as in the measurement of the area of absolute dulness (in which we measure only that portion of the heart which is uncovered by the lungs).

Hence, the changeability in the size of the heart, at least in slight grades, is ascertained with great difficulty. The changeability of the arterial pressure, on the other hand, is determined very easily by means of the sphygmomanometer. The fact that variations of arterial pressure in the same individual are readily detected with the sphygmomanometer is acknowledged by all investigators who use my instrument, even by those who deny that comparative study of the blood-pressure of different individuals can be made by its aid.

I do not agree with the latter opinion. I believe that the instrument will decide whether the blood-pressure of any individual is high or low. But in such cases we must be extremely careful and employ all the precautions recommended in my treatise on the sphygmomanometer.

For further information I may here add that, according to my experience, figures under 80 mm. Hg. indicate low pressure, those above 120 mm. Hg. high pressure. This is true of measurements upon the temporal artery. The values obtained upon the radial artery suffer from an error of 20 mm. Here figures under 100 mm. Hg. indicate low pressure, those above 140 mm. Hg. high pressure.

We have said that it is important in the diagnosis of cardiac dyspnœa to examine whether the size of the heart is changed and to determine the condition of the blood-pressure. The relations of blood-pressure to the diagnosis will be discussed later. We will first inquire whether the diagnosis of cardiac dyspnœa may be made when no change in the size of the heart is demonstrable. Without question. The area of cardiac dulness may be normal, the heart-sounds clear, and nevertheless cardiac dyspnœa may be present. In such cases and also in those in which there is a deviation from the normal, the diagnosis of pure cardiac dyspnœa, without complications, can only be made by exclusion. In other words, we must be able to show by the examination that the primary cause of the dyspnœa can only depend upon increase of pressure in the pulmonary artery. This can only be proven indirectly by the aid of measurement of the blood-pressure. When the dyspnœa results primarily from other conditions, which I have discussed in the introduction, we can no longer speak of pure cardiac dyspnœa.

Nevertheless the cardiac factor also plays a part in those cases in which the dyspnœa starts primarily from the lungs; when the elimination of a part of the respiratory surface by destructive processes impairs the respiratory capacity or when catarrhal swelling of the mucous membrane and accumulation of secretion in the bronchi interfere with the entrance of air, or when the loss of pulmonary elasticity prevents retraction of the lungs during expiration and consequently the respiratory interchange of gases is diminished.

In all these cases the dyspnœa is direct, *i.e.*, the imperfect respiration arises from diminished interchange of gases in the lungs themselves. This dyspnœa, or rather the induced dyspnœal condition of the blood, must give rise to increased arterial pressure and with it to increased rigidity of the lung. This rigidity has a so much greater injurious effect in all these cases because the interference with the respiratory capacity affects a lung whose function was already impaired.

It must also be remembered that in these pulmonary diseases the heart does not always remain healthy. Weakness of the heart is very often present in tuberculosis, but particularly in pneumonia, and emphysema is often associated with arterio-sclerosis and those diseases of the heart which arise from the nutritive disturbances due to arterio-sclerosis.

In order to obtain a better oversight, it is well to divide the cases of pure cardiac dyspnœa into two groups. In the first group, which includes the milder cases, dyspnœa does not occur until the pulmonary pressure is materially different from that present during the period of eupnœa. In these cases the irritant which produces the dyspnœa must be pronounced, or there must be marked irritability as a result of which a slight irritant is followed by a notable effect.

To express myself somewhat more concretely, we must include in this group those cases in which the increase of blood-pressure in the arteries and secondarily in the pulmonary artery only occurs after great bodily strain or in which a moderate exertion increases the blood-pressure very considerably. This category also includes the cases in which great increase of pressure readily occurs after excitement of a psychical character.

The heart and the circulation in general here present entirely normal conditions. The arterial pressure may be normal or deviate very little from the normal. Even low pressure may be observed, but this will not depend on pronounced cardiac weakness.

To this group belong the cases in which the dyspnœa is caused by obesity. This may be interpreted as an exciting cause only in so far as every bodily exertion which includes lifting the weight of the body, involves a relatively greater exertion. It also includes cases of anæmic irritable individuals who have a predisposition to palpitation of the heart, and finally cases of beginning arterio-sclerosis in which the arterial pressure is increased somewhat above the normal.

During the dyspnœa, examination shows, in these cases,

increased arterial pressure, enlargement of the lungs, and uniform enlargement of the heart.

In the second group, which includes the more severe cases, slight increase of pressure in the arteries or the pulmonary artery suffices to produce a degree of pulmonary rigidity which gives rise to dyspnœa. In these cases the stimulus which causes the dyspnœa is very slight, a trifling increase of bodily labor or mere change of position of the body. This will always occur when the pressure in the pulmonary artery has been relatively high from the start, either because the arterial pressure is very high or there is low arterial pressure due to permanent insufficiency of the heart.

In these cases the heart and circulation exhibit abnormal conditions. Either the arterial tension is very high and with it there is enlargement of the heart and probably hypertrophy, or the arterial tension is low and, at the same time, the right heart is larger than the left, and perhaps the pulmonary second sound accentuated. Distinct swelling, at times even pulsation, will be visible in the veins of the neck; swelling, dilatation, varicosities will also be found in other veins of the body.

This group includes cases of severe arterio-sclerosis without valvular lesion but with high arterial tension, cases of nephritis in which there is also high arterial tension, cases of arterio-sclerosis in every stage of the disease when the arterial pressure has fallen as the result of insufficiency of the heart, cases of general lipomatosis with weakness of the heart as the result of fatty degeneration of the heart muscle, and finally those cases of cardiac weakness which develop after acute infectious diseases, such as typhoid fever and diphtheria.

In these cases the arterial pressure will be found to be increased during the attack of dyspnœa. In cases of general cardiac hypertrophy, as in the first stages of arterio-sclerosis and in contracted kidneys, the enlargement of the heart during the dyspnœa will be general. When the increase of blood-pressure occurs in insufficiency of the heart, the right half probably undergoes greater enlargement than the left half. Distinct swelling or enlargement of the lungs can be demonstrated uniformly.

VI. Diagnosis of Cardiac Asthma.

As we have already remarked, the asthmatic attack is distinguished from dyspnœa chiefly by its suddenness. For this reason it was generally attributed to spasm. As the idea of spasm is always connected with the muscles, that form of asthma in which spasm of the bronchial muscular fibres or the diaphragm was assumed, has hitherto received more attention.

The term cardiac asthma has been restricted to those cases in which spasm of the diaphragm, bronchial muscles, or glottis can be excluded, and the causation is sought in the heart alone. All are agreed that suddenness does not distinguish nervous asthma with its different varieties from cardiac asthma. The sudden occurrence of cardiac asthma has not been explained hitherto. We have been satisfied with the notion that it is caused by cardiac failure. The small, feeble, barely perceptible pulse was regarded as the chief diagnostic sign. The answer to the question as to the explanation of the suddenness of cardiac asthma is no longer attended with difficulty.

Whoever has seen the lungs lose their distensibility at once after compression of the aorta or the injection of muscarin, will readily understand the suddenness of asthma. It is due to the rapidity with which the pulmonary rigidity develops.

We will hereafter consider the cardiac findings in the inter-paroxysmal period and will now discuss the attack itself from the diagnostic standpoint.

Two forms of asthma must be distinguished: 1, prodromal asthma; 2, asthma proper.

The diagnostic signs of prodromal asthma consist of great increase of the blood-pressure, *i.e.*, a very full, vigorous pulse, clearly demonstrable enlargement of the lungs as the result of swelling, and uniform enlargement of the heart.

The attack may consist solely of prodromal asthma and may subside as such. The prodromal asthma may also pass into asthma proper, and this transition may take place with more or less rapidity. It is attended with rapid fall of the blood-pressure, *i.e.*, with striking enfeeblement of the pulse.

Starting with the principles laid down in the section on "Pathology of Asthma," we must divide asthma proper into three varieties.

In the first variety the fall of blood-pressure is attended with that form of cardiac paresis in which the left ventricle mainly undergoes enlargement. The diagnostic signs, so far as regards the heart, are the following; the area of dulness increases on the left, and perhaps extends far beyond the mammary line. The apex-beat, more or less localized before the attack, becomes more diffuse and is superficial, undulating.

Toward the sternum the enlargement of the area of cardiac dulness is not demonstrable, and if it were present, the examination would show that it depends chiefly upon the left ventricle. The examination would have to take into consideration the difference between the sounds of the right and left heart rather than the area of dulness. As the action of the left heart is chiefly impaired, muffled, perhaps very feeble heart sounds would be heard over its entire area. This is true particularly of the first sound on account of the part played by muscular action in its production. If the dulness over the sternum corresponds to the left ventricle, then the muffled sounds of the left ventricle would be heard in that locality.

Over the right ventricle, whose action, on the whole, is very little changed and may even be intensified at a certain time, distinct sounds must be heard and there may even be temporary distinct accentuation of the second pulmonary sound.

In the second form of asthma proper, in which, according to my theory, the cardiac paresis that has caused lowering of the blood-pressure develops without relaxation and dilatation of the heart, and hence dilatation of the right ventricle, whose thin walls are more distensible, must develop, the dulness would first be increased toward the side of the sternum. But as distention of the left heart may increase the area of dulness on the right side, so distention of the right heart, when very marked, may also increase the dulness to the left, *i.e.*, beyond the mammary line. The question, whether the dulness on the left side belongs more to the right than to the left ventricle, must be decided by the careful examination of the heart sounds on the two sides. According to our assumption, the sounds over the right heart could not be so clearly distinguished by their intensity from the weaker sounds of the left heart. The apex-beat, in so far as it belongs to the left heart, would be weaker but not so diffuse as before; on the other hand, there would be strong epigastric pulsation starting from the right heart. Careful examination would also show considerable dulness in the region of the left auricle.

The third form of asthma proper could hardly be distinguished clinically from those just described, so far as regards the diagnostic signs referable to the heart, because dilatation of the right heart, and dilatation and fulness of the left auricle, would be characteristic phenomena. This variety would only be distinguished from the others by the etiological element, *i.e.*, by the cardiac spasm which induces the changes mentioned.

The diagnostic signs of the last two forms of asthma just furnished, apart from their theoretical foundation upon experiments on animals, are by no means so hypothetical as we might believe. The literature contains a number of cases in which the same diagnostic signs which we have deduced from experiments, are described. The most pertinent one is the case of sudden asthma observed by Albutt upon himself and carefully described. On account of its importanec I will here quote literally. "I was attacked quite suddenly by a strange and peculiar want of breath, accompanied by an extremely disagreeable sensation of fulness and pulsation in the epigastrium. On placing my hand upon my heart I felt a labored diffuse beat over the entire epigastrium. I opened my shirt at once and convinced myself by percussion that the right ventricle was dilated very considerably. I therefore threw myself upon the grass at full length with the shoulders raised, and in a few minutes enjoyed the satisfaction of finding that the dilatation of the heart, the oppression, and the cardiac dulness were diminishing. I was then able to rise and sit down and even to walk on the level, but the symptoms returned as soon as I began to ascend."

Stokes describes, in his well-known work on Diseases of the Heart, a case of sudden dilatation of the left auricle in an attack of cardiac asthma. Barié (quoted in Fraenkel's article on Asthma in Eulenburg's Encyclopædia) speaks of dyspeptic asthma in which, according to him, the right heart is enlarged; in this case the cardiac dulness was increased to the left, and this circumstance led Fraenkel to believe that the right heart was not enlarged. But as Barié expressly emphasizes the accentuation of the second pulmonary sound, his opinion that he had to deal with enlargement of the right heart was probably more correct. The direction of dulness alone does not decide the question whether the right or left heart takes the greater part in the enlargement.

I concede willingly that the clinical observations are too few to permit us to base upon them alone the theory of spasm or retraction of the heart. But a theory which is founded firmly on experiment and is supported by post-mortem findings, a theory which is supported even by a few clinical observations, is not founded on air and must be taken into consideration in clinical observations. I have no doubt that what has been seen in rare cases by a few excellent observers will be seen more frequently. That these observations should be so rare is not astonishing. Patients suffering from cardiac asthma are very rarely seen during an attack, especially when they occur at night. Even when they are seen during the seizure, the chief attention is directed to the threatening symptoms—the pulse is felt and the heart auscultated, but only in order to ascertain its general condition. The lungs are auscultated in order to determine whether œdema is beginning, but careful examination is omitted, as a rule, in order to spare the patient. But when the path of examination is mapped out more strictly, there will soon, I hope, be no dearth of observations which will inform us concerning the condition of the heart during asthma, and it is to be expected that these observations will be in harmony with the few already made and with the theories here advanced.

In the last two forms of cardiac asthma the pulse is less tense, corresponding with the diminished arterial pressure. In the spasmodic form, if there be such a form, the soft pulse would be larger than in the paretic form. I deduce this sign from experiment; clinical observation must show whether it holds good.

In all three forms of asthma, swelling or enlargement of the lungs must be demonstrable.

Enlargement of the lungs during an attack of asthma has been regarded hitherto as the most important sign of bronchial asthma. The occlusion of the finest bronchi—whether from spasm, acute catarrh or bronchiolitis, as assumed lately, was supposed to act like a valve, which permits the entrance of air but interferes with its exit. In this way it was sup-

posed that more air would be stored in the alveoli and distend
the lungs. In accordance with this, the percussion sound in
bronchial asthma approaches the tympanitic character, and
Biermer's so-called " box " sound is heard on percussion.

I do not wish to enter upon the theory of bronchial asthma;
but, in my opinion, enlargement of the lung as such can no
longer be attributed solely to occlusion of the bronchi. From
the standpoint of differential diagnosis, the enlargement can
no longer be regarded as pathognomonic of bronchial asthma.
But it is possible that the distended lung of bronchial asthma
is distinguished by the " box " sound from that of cardiac
asthma.

The most important distinctions between the two conditions must be sought—apart from the etiological factors, *i.e.,*
previous catarrh of the bronchi—in the results of auscultation
during the asthma and in the character of the respiration.
In cardiac asthma no abnormal respiratory murmurs are
heard, so long as œdema of the lungs does not develop. The
respiration is feeble, as a rule, and coarse râles are heard only
at the close of the attack. When œdema occurs during the
attack, distinct crepitant râles are heard and it is often possible to demonstrate slight dulness in places. In cardiac asthma
the dyspnœa is general, *i.e.,* mixed; both inspiration and expiration are prolonged and labored. All observers agree that
the respiration is slowed, not accelerated.

In bronchial asthma, auscultation shows numerous obstruc-
tions to the entrance and exit of air, which are recognized by
the whistling, rattling, wheezing, and numerous rhonchi. The
striking feature is the difficult expiration, which is attended
with loud, high-pitched, sighing sounds, and distinct strain of
the expiratory muscles.

Two years ago I had the opportunity of seeing an attack
of pronounced bronchial asthma and of measuring the blood-
pressure during the attack. The pressure was increased to a
very high degree. Measured at the radial artery the pressure
usually amounted to 150 mm. mercury, but during the attack
it rose to 200 mm. This great increase was undoubtedly produced by the dyspnœa which was due in turn to the impeded
respiration.

Can a bronchial asthma, which is attended with increase of
blood-pressure, be regarded as pure bronchial asthma? I

think not. The increased pressure must give rise to pulmonary rigidity and, if we assume that the bronchial asthma began only with dilatation of the alveoli, then, when the dyspnœa in the course of the attack increases the blood-pressure, swelling and rigidity of the lungs must develop. In other words, bronchial asthma under high arterial pressure is no longer a pure bronchial asthma, but is a combination of this form with prodromal cardiac asthma.

In every attack of bronchial asthma in which we find a full, very tense pulse, we must therefore make the diagnosis of this combined condition. It is very probable that bronchial asthma is also combined with cardiac asthma proper, and this will be the case when the pulse is small and feeble during the attack.

The predisposition to cardiac asthma depends only in slight part upon the condition of the lungs during the inter-paroxysmal period. We observe attacks occasionally in individuals who suffer from more or less severe emphysema, and I have also observed it in a case of pulmonary phthisis, but the condition also occurs in individuals whose lungs are otherwise perfectly normal.

Dyspeptic asthma belongs in the front rank of those forms of cardiac asthma in which the lungs are perfectly normal.

This variety is decidedly a cardiac asthma and is so regarded by Fraenkel in his article in Eulenburg's Encyclopædia. Henoch has called special attention to this form and explains it by the experiments of Mayer and Pribram which showed that distention of the stomach increases the blood-pressure and irritates the central ends of the pneumogastric. The relations of these experiments to dyspeptic asthma have become much clearer since I have shown, from a new standpoint, the part played by increase of blood-pressure in dyspnoea and asthma. We now easily understand how dyspnœa or a prodromal asthma is produced by distention of the stomach and intestines, if this has been followed by increased blood-pressure. As is easily seen, the two most important conditions for its development are here combined, viz., the pulmonary rigidity and swelling as the result of the increased blood-pressure, and the respiratory insufficiency due to elevation of the diaphragm.

Dyspeptic asthma will remain a prodromal asthma so long

as it is associated with high blood-pressure. It may also be converted into asthma proper when the heart falls from its condition of equilibrium in any of the ways mentioned above. As in the experiments of Mayer and Pribram, the slowing of the pulse may also occur during dyspeptic asthma in its pro-dromal stage and for the same reasons. This slowing of the pulse may be absent in the second stage in which the blood-pressure is lower, and even acceleration of the pulse may occur at this time.

Barié's case favors the view that, in dyspeptic asthma, the heart passes out of the condition of equilibrium in that form in which there is dilatation of the right heart.

It must be left undecided whether the distention of the stomach and intestines produces asthma merely in a reflex manner, *i.e.*, by irritation of the vaso-motor centres; or whether a condition of paralysis or irritation of the diaphragm is not produced in another reflex manner as in the act of vom-iting, which is associated with spasm of the diaphragm and the expiratory muscles; or whether a part is not played by toxic influences as the result of absorption of gastric and in-testinal gases or of ptomaines developing in the contents of the digestive canal and which might possibly act like mus-carin.

As is well known, dyspeptic asthma subsides with eructa-tions or passage of intestinal gases. It is questionable whether the diminished tension of the stomach and intestines or the escape of the gases in a chemical sense plays the prin-cipal part.

In many cases, uræmic asthma is undoubtedly a pure car-diac asthma. In individuals who suffer from nephritis, the arterial tension is very high, as a rule, and hence the predis-position to asthma is very great. Prodromal asthma as well as asthma proper are very apt to develop. If we take into consideration that pulmonary œdema develops very often in such cases, we might be led to infer that paretic retraction or spasm of the heart is most apt to occur here, because these forms favor the production of œdema of the lungs. But it must also be taken into consideration that the hydræmic con-dition of the blood may favor the transudation of fluid into the alveoli.

The increased transudation from hydræmic blood causes

the development of cerebral œdema in these cases. This œdema may act secondarily upon the heart, by irritation of the central origin of the vaso-motor or cardiac nerves, and thus indirectly on the lungs. The coma, which sometimes occurs during the asthmatic attack, is connected with the œdema. It cannot be denied, however, that toxic influences due to the retention of certain substances in the blood may play a part in uræmia, and possibly give rise to the asthma or coma.

Attacks of asthma have also been observed in a few cases of lead poisoning. As the arterial tension is very high in lead poisoning, it may be assumed that we have to deal here with cardiac asthma. The causes for the development of the latter are present in the same manner as in arterio-sclerosis and nephritis.

In the inter-paroxysmal period we must examine the condition of the heart, pulse and lungs with regard to the diagnosis, and may classify the cases into groups.

The first group includes cases of arterio-sclerosis and aortic lesions due to sclerotic changes. These are characterized by enlargement of the heart, especially of the left ventricle, and a high tension pulse. Cases of nephritis, in which attacks of cardiac asthma occur, also belong to this group.

The second group inludes cases of low arterial tension and valvular lesions of the left venous orifice. Here the enlargement of the heart, when present, will affect chiefly the right side of the heart.

As regards the anatomical diagnosis, we may only speak of fatty heart (in which the function of the heart muscle has suffered in a notable degree) in those cases of the second group in which the blood-pressure is very low, excluding those in which considerable lesions of the mitral valve cause the slight filling of the arterial system. In the cases of the first group we may assume those changes in the structure of the heart which result from arterio-sclerosis.

"Special attention must be paid to the condition of the lungs because from this we must decide whether the attack is pure cardiac asthma or a mixed form of cardiac and bronchial asthma. If catarrh is demonstrable in the lungs or bronchi, we must ascertain whether it is primarily pulmonary in character or only a sequel of those circulatory disturbances which

lead to the dyspnœa or cardiac asthma. As a rule, this question cannot be answered by a single examination, but only by
continued observation, the success or failure of therapeutic
measures being also taken into consideration."

Nor is it easy to decide whether a demonstrable enlargement of the lung is due to true emphysema. In this regard
we must always remember that high arterial tension as such
causes swelling of the lung, and that the possibility of high
pressure in the pulmonary artery and hence pulmonary swelling must be thought of even when the arterial tension is not
high. The differential diagnosis between pulmonary swelling
—perhaps Traube's volumen pulmonum auctum also belongs
here—and pulmonary emphysema is therefore worthy of more
consideration. The emphysema may be demonstrated on
autopsy; whether this is true of swelling of the lungs must be
determined by future investigations.

Theoretical considerations seem to show that emphysema
probably constitutes a constant condition, pulmonary swelling
a variable condition during life.

VII. Course and Terminations of Cardiac Dyspnœa and Cardiac Asthma.

Cardiac dyspnœa ceases with the cessation of the causes
that have produced it, *i.e.*, in bodily rest or changed position
of the body. Prodromal asthma may also subside spontaneously when the blood-pressure sinks.

This spontaneous lowering of the blood-pressure can only
be explained by the notion that the irritation of the vaso-
motor centre, after it has lasted a long time, diminishes on
account of exhaustion, and that the vessels of the greater circulation dilate as the result of this diminished irritability,
despite the existing dyspnœa. With the increased flow of
blood from the left heart the pulmonary vessels will also be
emptied, the pulmonary rigidity will diminish in a corresponding measure, the distensibility of the lungs becomes greater,
the dyspnœic respiratory movements cause thorough ventilation of the blood, and the dyspnœic blood is thus converted
into eupnœic blood. As a matter of course, the attack then
subsides.

In asthma proper, the power of the heart must be increased

before the attack will subside. The patient instinctively attempts to intensify the heart's action by bodily movement or changed position of the body (in Stokes' well-known case the patient bent his head to the ground and thus escaped the attack). Such procedures sometimes abort the attack. The exhaustion of the vaso-motor centre or the dilatation of the vessels may also act favorably, in so far as this entails the more ready passage of the blood from the lungs. As a matter of course, this can only occur when the paresis of the heart is not very marked.

As regards the sequelæ of dyspnœa and asthma, it must be kept in mind that the dyspnœic blood, on account of its poverty in oxygen, has an unfavorable influence upon the heart. The nutrition of the organ, which is frequently traversed by the dyspnœic blood, must be affected unfavorably, and as the insufficiency of oxygen favors fatty degeneration of the albumin, according to A. Fraenkel's experiment, frequently recurring dyspnœa or asthma may give rise to fatty degeneration of the heart. Unfavorable nutritive conditions also arise from the fact that the nutrient vessels of the heart and rest of the body are narrowed by the dyspnœa, so that the amount of blood supply is also changed unfavorably in every dyspnœa or asthma.

In addition to the direct injury to the heart muscle, the repeated increase of intracardial pressure distends the heart muscle and, as a result, there may be permanent malformation (dilatation of one or both ventricles).

VIII. TREATMENT.

IN the treatment of different affections which have one cardinal symptom in common—in our case dyspnœa—individualization is only possible when we have clear conceptions of the physiological character of the affection in each individual case. But the most important part is played by experience because it alone can inform us concerning the true value of the conceptions by which we are guided in treatment.

In this manner I will discuss the treatment of the affections under consideration.

In the milder cases we must pay the chief attention to the causal indication, because we start with the assumption that

the heart itself is sound. Here the increase of the weight of
the body is the principal cause of the dyspnœal symptoms and
its reduction is the most important object of treatment. This
reduction should be confined, if possible, to that tissue whose
overgrowth is useless or even injurious to the body and necessitates superfluous work in locomotion. The question simply
is, How is the excess best removed, what mode of reducing
obesity is the best? The principle is simple: increase the consumption of fat and spare the albuminoid substances.

The consumption of fat is attended by processes which furnish carbonic acid and water as final products, when these
processes furnish the material from which the final products
are obtained. These processes include particularly increased
muscular effort and production of heat. The stored-up fat
must supply the material for these processes when the carbohydrates, ingested in the food, no longer suffice. The albumin
of the body is saved from loss when the deprivation of carbohydrates is not carried too far. All modes of treatment of
obesity, whatever may be their name, vary within these limits.

Simple as these requirements may appear from a theoretical standpoint, it is difficult to meet them in the individual
case.

A rational procedure requires that, in the individual case,
we ask whether the chief importance should be attached to an
increase of the processes which stimulate consumption or to a
diminution of fat-producing food.

Under certain circumstances measures which meet the first
requirement will suffice. It is often found that a few pedes-
trian trips suffice to reduce the weight of the body by a few
kilogrammes. Hence, when there is no special indication, we
may simply recommend increased exercise to obese individuals
who begin to complain of dyspnœa. In giving this injunction,
however, we must always consider the habits of the individual
and avoid a sudden transition to others. This rule is clear if
we remember that we are unable to gauge properly the effect
of such sudden transitions. The increased exercise must not
degenerate into hard work which is followed by exhaustion,
and special care is to be taken that the condition which we
desire to remove by the exercise, viz., the dyspnœa, is not increased by the exercise itself. As we have mentioned above,
dyspnœa always indicates the presence of a poor quality of

blood, imperfect filling of the capillaries, over-distention of the veins, and thus an unfavorable nutritive condition of the body. The frequent return of such a condition can hardly fail to be attended by permanent bad effects.

The increase of bodily work may be recommended in various ways. The simplest is to direct the patient to walk more. At first he should walk upon the level, but he may pass gradually to climbing.

The subjective sensations of the patient are the only measure of the sufficiency of the exercise. We may, however, give directions as regards the duration of the exercise. We may begin with one to two hours and then increase to six hours, sometimes even more. The distance to be traversed in the time mentioned must always be left to the patient himself.

No objection is to be made to Scholl's recommendation to begin with light gymnastics, provided we are convinced that it does not produce a greater strain than mere walking. But it must be remembered that gymnastic exercises produce a much greater effect, because larger groups of muscles, which are usually not employed vigorously, are then brought into action. Gymnastic exercises, which effect distention of the thorax, are undoubtedly useful in improving respiration. This I observed in my service at the Policlinic in a young man who had formerly suffered a good deal from palpitation of the heart and difficulty in breathing; both symptoms disappeared after he engaged in rowing. Inspection showed that the pectorals were remarkably well developed in this otherwise feeble individual.

As already mentioned, the consumption of the bodily fat is increased during muscular work, if the introduction of carbohydrates is diminished at the same time.

The extent to which we must go in this direction cannot be determined before treatment. At all events the plan for the changed diet must be formed in accordance with the previous mode of life of the patient and the condition of his digestion. Very often almost no change in the diet can be made. In many cases, on the other hand, very decided changes may be made in the amount and constitution of the food.

Dietetic treatment should never be carried to excess, and to define the limits in this direction is one of the most difficult problems in the treatment of obesity.

In accordance with the principles laid down in prescribing bodily exercise, I also plead here for mild methods. I am no friend of so-called vigorous treatment. As a matter of experience, the latter does not effect very much in reducing the weight.

How often have I seen that, among different patients of apparently similar constitution, the weight of one diminished more than three times that of the other. When the latter, envious of the brilliant results of treatment in the former, imposed upon himself the greatest possible abstinence, it was found that he grew only weaker, but not materially lighter than before. The effect obtained was disproportionate to the abstinence and, what is most important, to the injurious effects whose real extent cannot be measured. Scholl has properly called attention to the dangers which may arise from over-treatment of obesity.

The question of diet has been discussed so much of late years that it may seem superfluous to say anything further. The general principles are quite firmly established, their execution must be regulated by the physician and patient in each individual case.

In the last few years deprivation of fluids has been recommended in addition to reduction of the carbohydrates. This advice is based on the idea that the diminished ingestion of fluids diminishes the amount of blood in circulation and that such diminution is capable of relieving the dyspnœa. I have already shown that weighty objections may be raised against this view. According to the new theory of cardiac asthma which I have here advanced and which can only be overthrown by proving that my data are wrong, this idea must be regarded as erroneous. In favor of this reduction of fluid can only be mentioned its supposed results in practice and the increase of the renal secretion which, according to Feilchenfeld's corroborative experiment, it is said to have. The practical results, however, have been denied by various observers. As regards the increase of the urinary secretion, it is by no means clear upon what it depends and what it signifies. It is very possible that the increased secretion of urine after deprivation of fluid indicates a condition similar to diabetes insipidus. At all events, the contrary has not been proven.

The loss of fat can also be aided considerably by the internal use of waters containing Glauber's salts and sodium chloride (Marienbad, Tarasp, Karlsbad, Kissingen, etc.). So far as I can judge from my own experience, waters containing Glauber's salt are admirably adapted to this purpose. It can very often be noted with certainty that their use diminishes the weight of the body even when the consumption of fat has not been increased by exercise, and the improvement may even be observed when there has been no restriction in diet.

Baths (carbonated, brine and vapor baths) are also therapeutic aids in this direction, because they stimulate the nutritive processes, increase the production of carbonic acid, and the urinary and cutaneous secretions.

Increased exercise may also be useful in those mild cases without demonstrable changes in the cardiac function, and in which the increased weight of the body due to the abundance of adipose cannot be regarded as the exciting cause. The cause of improvement is not to be sought in the reduction of weight, because this is not even desirable here, but in other circumstances. Among these, habit occupies the first rank. We can readily conceive that in individuals who lead a too quiet life, either for extrinsic reasons or because they feel too weak, a slight excess of movement will produce dyspnœa and that in consequence of the muscular rest there develops an increased sensibility to the dyspnœal stimuli produced by muscular exertion; in addition, the muscular respiratory apparatus, which has become lazy, loses its regulating capacity. In such cases exercise secures the therapeutic objects of blunting the sensibility and of stimulating the regulating capacity of the respiratory mechanism. Walking and cautious, progressively increasing climbing constitute respiratory gymnastics in such cases and it is also advantageous to pay special attention to the muscles of the thorax. This form of dyspnœa is found in young anæmic and chlorotic individuals and also in neurasthenics.

The dyspnœa of chlorotic and anæmic individuals has been associated by various writers (Sée, Brunton) with the imperfect ability of the blood to take up oxygen. Such a condition of the blood really favors dyspnœa in so far as every muscular effort, when the absorption of oxygen is diminished, signifies a relative increase of the carbonic acid, *i.e.*, an increase of the dyspnæal irritation of the blood. But the dyspnœa of anæmia and chlorosis is, in reality, a cardiac dyspnœa. This view is in harmony with the fact that, in such cases, we often find a tendency to palpitation which is probably dependent on the dyspnœal irritation of the vascular system that is apt to occur, and that, as I have observed in a number of cases, is followed by increase of blood-pressure. [Perhaps this fact also stands in causal relation to the tendency to cardiac hypertrophy in such cases to which Sée has called special attention.]

Bodily exercise also has another object, viz., to secure permanent increase, if possible, of the heart's action. This is particularly indicated when measurement shows the existence of very low blood-pressure.

In such cases we must overcome the opposition of the patient to walking and insist upon it even when it is connected with slight dyspnœa. This sends more blood to the heart than usual, and, as a matter of experience, it is found that the dyspnœa is soon overcome by the more vigorous respiration. The diet should be stimulating. Wine and beer are to be recommended in these cases, despite the dyspnœa and the vascular changes which often produce congestions. If there is a tendency to obesity this must be taken into consideration, as a matter of course, in prescribing diet. The internal administration of iron and arsenic is often useful. When the blood-pressure appeared to be especially low, I have used strychnine or tincture of nux vomica with success. Lukewarm baths— carbonated iron baths and mud baths—are auxiliary remedies.

Whether the dyspnœa of neurasthenics is cardiac in character, cannot be ascertained with certainty. The cardiac factor undoubtedly plays an important part in certain cases in which great irritability of the vascular system and heart is demonstrable. Such cases must be treated with great caution. The condition of the patients is sometimes improved by bodily exercise, sometimes it is made worse. When the dyspnœa is produced not alone by movement, but is also noticed during rest, as the need of taking deep breath frequently, medicinal treatment is also indicated. I have seen some good results from strychnine and nitroglycerin. Neurasthenics react in a different manner to baths as they do to exercise. Mild cold-water cures sometimes act favorably, but cold is often tolerated poorly. In the latter event it is advisable to try lukewarm baths. Neurasthenics are sometimes very sensitive to baths containing carbonic acid; mud baths are tolerated much better.

In the severer cases of dyspnœa which are due to demonstrable valvular lesions or to supposed structural changes in the heart as shown by functional changes, special attention must be paid in treatment—apart from the data furnished by examination of the heart—to the results of measurement of the blood-pressure or the condition of the pulse.

As regards immediate interference, it is not immaterial whether we have to deal with a patient with high arterial pressure, *i.e.,* a high tension pulse, or low arterial pressure, *i.e.,* a soft pulse. It is also very important to note the change of blood-pressure uninterruptedly during the course of treatment.

We will first consider those cases in which the arterial pressure has been found to be high, *i.e.,* those in which there is very probably arterio-sclerosis or valvular lesions as the result of arterio-sclerosis.

So far as regards treatment, we must here distinguish between cases which are associated with obesity and those in which arterio-sclersois is unattended with this anomaly of nutrition or is even combined with distinct emaciation.

Cases of arterio-sclerosis with general lipomatosis, so long as the vascular tension does not exceed the normal to a great extent, are subject to the same principles of treatment as simple obesity. These are the cases which usually figure in practice under the head of abdominal plethora.

Cautious exercise and moderate regimen for obesity will play the chief part; and special aid is derived from the therapeutic measures which give rise to derivation. Care must be taken to secure copious evacuations from the bowels, if necessary by the use of purgatives. The abdominal cavity is thus reduced in size and the intra-abdominal pressure diminished. This aids in diminishing the arterial pressure. With the lowering of the pressure in the arteries the swelling and rigidity of the lung will also diminish. The distention of the lungs becomes easier and respiration may become more free, especially when, on account of the evacuation of the bowels, the excursions of the diaphragm are no longer interfered with and the weight of the body has diminished under treatment. The favorable effect of those mineral water cures, which stimulate the evacuation of the bowels, undoubtedly depends on this action. Traube called attention repeatedly to the importance of purgation in arterio-sclerosis. Nevertheless, this important factor in the treatment of certain circulatory disturbances has been undervalued of late years; and some writers even warn against the use of purgatives. It is true that the continued use of strong purgatives may be injurious to the intestines, and may give rise to chronic catarrh with increasing atony of the muscular coat of the intestines. The latter condition is combated less easily than the former and leads to the necessity of administering progressively increasing doses.

But if, in cases in which the tension of the pulse is high, we reflect which is the lesser injury, the high tension and its effects upon the heart, circulation, respiration, etc., or the injurious after-effect of purgatives, we will hardly waver in an our choice and will continue purgation. In my experience, moreover, the after-effects of purgatives are not so injurious as is generally believed. I know individuals who for years have taken aloes daily and feel perfectly well. As a rule, purgatives are not injurious until their action begins to flag. In the same way, as I know by experience at Marienbad, the use of saline laxative waters is injurious only so long as they do not purge, however abundant the urinary secretion may be. Under such circumstances the patients complain of labored breathing, distended abdomen, loss of appetite, rush of blood to the head, etc.

The use of baths, in these cases, possesses the advantage of increasing the consumption of fat. But on account of the injury which may accrue from any increase of the blood-pressure, we must convince ourselves by tests whether any reaction, which points to such an increase, becomes noticeable immediately after the beginning of the bath, during or after the bath. There is no doubt that baths may act as a stimulant. In a case of this kind I measured the blood-pressure and found it considerably higher than in the patient's normal condition. Such an elevation has little significance in individuals with a weak pulse, but it is important in cases in which the tension of the pulse is already higher than normal. Warm baths may also act in a decidedly favorable manner in such cases by dilating the cutaneous vessels and, in a reflex way, the abdominal vessels, and thus diminishing the pressure in the aorta. Whether this is also true of vapor baths or whether they do not rather give rise to considerable elevation of blood-pressure, I do not know and on this account I avoid ordering vapor baths in cases of arterio-sclerosis. Nor do I regard cold baths as indicated, on account of their action in increasing the blood-pressure. Cases have been reported in which violent dyspnœal symptoms developed after cold baths and even increased to asthma. Such cases also warn us to be cautious.

In cases of arterio-sclerosis in which obesity is not present, we dispense with those therapeutic measures which are intended for the consumption of fat, and it only appears necessary to bring the pulse into a condition of the lowest possible tension. This is effected chiefly, as we have already said, by the use of purgatives. When these have produced relief, a diet must be maintained which prevents the accumulation of fæcal masses as much as possible, viz., a milk and meat diet, no leguminous or farinaceous food, but especially no potatoes. In such cases the urinary secretion is more abundant than usual and there is no reason for therapeutic interference in this direction.

Alcoholic drinks, in large amounts, are contraindicated for the reason that alcoholism is known to be one of the causes of arterio-sclerosis. But it is not advisable to deprive the patients entirely, especially when they are advanced in years, of the use of alcohol in the form of wine or beer.

All forms of excessive exercise must be carefully avoided. The patient may be allowed moderate exercise, if it can be performed without dyspnœa; occupations attended with bodily strain must be interdicted.

In addition to purgatives and suitable dietetic regimen, we may also resort, when necessary, to cardiac remedies. One of the mildest of these, according to my experience, is atropine in very small doses. My prescription reads: sol. atropiæ sulph. (0.3%), 1.0, aq. destill. 150.0, one tablespoonful every three to five hours. Formerly I used atropia only in arhythmia, starting with the physiological notion that it made the heart insensible to irritation of the vagus. I then found that it also acts favorably upon dyspnœa and have since employed it when arhythmia as not present. I have obtained good results in my service at the Policlinic and also in my private practice in

Marienbad. Atropine I have used only for a year; formerly I gave the extract or tincture of belladonna, the former in doses of 0.01 p. d., the latter five to six drops p. d.

When atropine alone is unsuccessful, we should resort to digitalis. In former years, on the basis of theoretical considerations, I regarded the high tension of the pulse as a contra-indication to the use of digitalis. I was strengthened in this opinion because my sphygmomanometric measurements showed that in cases of low tension of the pulse, in which I used digitalis, the improvement of the respiratory disturbances was often associated with increasing arterial pressure.

Experience has taught me, in opposition to this opinion, that digitalis sometimes acts favorably when it is used in cases with high tension pulse. Such a result involves no contradiction, but is rather to be expected on closer study. High arterial tension does not exclude, as I have already shown, a high tension in the venous system and the lesser circulation. Therapeutically, however, we have to deal much more with the removal of the two latter symptoms. If, as may be assumed, digitalis is able to do this, then its good effects are readily explained. Hence the indication for the use of digitalis resides, in my opinion, not so much in the condition of arterial pressure as it does in that of the venous pressure. When there are signs of the increase of the latter—swelling or pulsation of the cervical veins—digitalis should be administered. It is particularly indicated when high arterial pressure gradually diminishes with the increasing dyspnœa and when greater swelling or pulsation of the cervical veins sets in, because this is due undoubtedly to diminished activity of the heart. When the arterial tension is very high constantly or exhibits a tendency to increase still more, it is questionable whether digitalis should be given.

For some time I have been in the habit of giving digitalis in combination with atropine, 1 gm. of 0.3% solution of atropine being added to 150.0 of an infusion of varying strengths. In a series of mild as well as severe cases and also in cases of severe valvular lesions, I have convinced myself that digitalis, with this addition, is well borne for a long time. In the comparative tests which I made, it seemed as if the combination of digitalis and atropine had a better effect on the heart than digitalis alone. I may take this opportunity of remarking that this form of medication is also based on experimental experience. Experiment shows that the injection of such a mixed solution into the jugular of a dog produces an increase of blood-pressure which apparently lasts longer than that produced by infusion of digitalis alone. A striking feature in this experiment was the condition of the venous pressure, which fell materially despite the high and constant increase of arterial pressure.

In such cases I also order lobelia in addition to atropine and digitalis. I prescribe a mixture containing 2 to 3 gms. tinct. lobeliæ to 150.0 water and add to this 1 gm. of the 0.3% solution of atropine. I have observed a number of cases in which this treatment was followed by tolerably favorable results.

The cases in which examination with the sphygmomanometer shows very high tension—in my experience such cases have a radial tension of 180–200 mm. Hg.—must be treated with special caution. If obesity is also present, we must attempt to reduce the weight by suitable diet. The urine must always be examined for albumin in these cases. When it is not found, we may attempt to reduce the ingestion of fluids as much as possible. On account of the rigidity and unyielding character of the walls of the vessels it is possible that the increased absorption of fluid may lead to increase of blood-pressure, and this, however slight, is to be avoided at any cost. When albumin is present in the urine, we must avoid excessive reduction of fluids because the danger of producing uræmia artificially by such means is not excluded.

As the lungs are already swollen[1] on account of the enormous increase of the blood-pressure and hence dyspnœa occurs from very slight causes and very moderate exercise, we may only permit walking on the level at the beginning of treatment. Climbing should be allowed only after noticeable improvement has occurred. As a matter of course, purgation is more important in such cases than in others. I am in the habit of giving atropine when irregularity of the heart's action (arhythmia) is demonstrable, also in the galop rhythm and

---

[1] I have recently demonstrated this enlargement of the lungs in an exquisite case. The patient was a very stout man, aged 40 years, weight of body 150 kg.; severe dyspnœa on walking. Examination showed transposition of the lungs over the heart; bruit de rapelle. Pressure in the radial artery 190 mm. Hg.

bruit de rapelle. This irregularity sometimes depends upon the high tension under which the heart is acting (this is confirmed by well-known experiments on animals) and may disappear spontaneously with the diminution of pressure. But atropine often aids materially in securing uniformity of the heart's action. The arhythmia does not disappear at once but gradually. As a general thing, the type first changes, the complete irregularity is converted into allorhythmia, *i.e.*, a form of arhythmia which occurs with a certain degree of regularity (bigemini, trigemini). The most important factor in judging the form of arhythmia is not so much the rhythm of the pulse, *i.e.*, the varying duration of the individual beats and the varying intervals between them, but rather the variability in the strength of the different beats. On the whole, this can be detected very well with the finger, although a better insight is afforded by measurement of the blood-pressure with the sphygmomanometer. This informs us concerning the differences of arterial pressure during the periods of the larger and smaller pulse beats. Hence the measurement is a much more certain gauge than the finger of the degree of arhythmia. The greater the difference between the maximum and minimum pressure, as shown by the instrument, the greater is the arhythmia and its injurious influence. Sphygmomanometric measurement will show that the differences between the maximum and minimum become less, despite the persistence of arhythmia, and this is a distinct indication that the latter has improved despite its persistence. This is found not infrequently after the use of atropine and also when the drug is combined with digitalis. The difference is reduced to a minimum, so that the pulse merely remains irregular, and even the irregularity may disappear. I may here remark that intermissions of the pulse resist treatment more obstinately than arhythmia. However, many cases are found in which the latter symptom also resists every plan of treatment.

I am not in the habit of giving digitalis in such cases or, at least, only when an exacerbation occurs, attended with lowering of the blood-pressure. I have sometimes tried sodium iodide, according to Huchard's recommendation. No striking diminution of arterial tension was observed after the administration of this remedy. It is well tolerated even after prolonged use and appears to diminish the tendency to dyspnœa in certain cases.

What are the principles according to which those cases, in which the dyspnœa is attended with weak heart's action, are to be treated? Undoubtedly the chief object of treatment must be to remove the cardiac weakness as far as possible. The treatment of the individual case must therefore be preceded by the consideration of the factors to which the development of the cardiac weakness may be attributed.

The occurrence of weak heart in obese individuals is explained very easily because it is evident that the general nutritive disturbance must also affect the heart muscle, and may thus give rise to fatty degeneration and weakness of the heart. Due attention must therefore be paid to the general disturbance of nutrition in these cases, as well as in those in which obesity is attended with high arterial tension. The consumption of fat offers the possibility of the disappearance of the adipose tissue situated upon the heart and between its muscular fibres. The reduction of weight acts favorably by diminishing the muscular effort necessary to raise the body, and also diminishes the dyspnœal irritants produced by muscular effort.

The same rules hold good here as formerly in the treatment of obesity, except that bodily exercise possesses even greater importance. Here the exercise not alone increases the consumption of fat, but also effects another important object, viz., thorough filling of the left heart. the arteries and capillaries of the greater circulation.

In conditions of heart weakness, the distribution of blood is gradually changed, so that the veins are filled more abundantly at the cost of the arteries and capillaries. Inasmuch as the vis a tergo of the feeble left ventricle is slight, the blood flows slowly from the dilated veins into the right ventricle, and the latter does not fill the pulmonary vessels under high pressure unless the pressure in the left auricle has increased on account of the accumulation of blood which the left ventricle could not expel into the arteries. So long as the blood flows from the pulmonary vessels into the left auricle without any material obstruction, it may be assumed that dyspnœa will not occur. This will only develop when, as the result of increasing pressure in the left auricle, the capillaries of the pulmonary alveoli are brought under greater tension. The increasing pressure in the left auricle is the direct result of the insufficiency of the feeble heart, but this is only manifested distinctly when the heart is called upon to do increased work which it cannot meet completely, *i.e.*, when the heart must evacuate its contents under great resistance. This is particn-larly true of the left ventricle because this is first subjected to the influence of the variations in resistance which are so apt to occur in the greater circulation. Such variations act only in an indirect manner upon the right heart.

If bodily exercise is increased to such an extent that strong stimuli (which do not, however, exceed physiological limits) are produced, then these stimuli induce more powerful or deeper respiratory movements. The latter offer favorable conditions for the accelerated flow of blood from the veins toward the thorax, for greater distention of the arteries and capillaries of the body and, what is very important, for the greater fulness of the nutrient arteries of the heart. As a matter of course, the increased fulness of the heart may only be permitted to proceed to the extent to which the heart is still capable of accommodation. The over-stepping of this limit is manifested at once by severe dyspnœa.

Favorable as is the increased fulness of the heart, with the associated increased action and increased passage of blood through its coronary arteries, its over-distention is equally in-jurions. Over-distention of an insufficient heart must give rise to dyspnœa because the organ is incapable of the work which is necessary to throw into the greater circulation the blood that has entered the thoracic organs as the result of the deep inspirations.

In the cases which are now under consideration, the thera-peutic rule may be established that movement of the body should only be permitted to that extent at which the necessity arises for breathing more deeply and rapidly. Even at this point there is certainly an increase of the arterial pressure, but it is merely an expression of moderate distention of the left ventricle and is therefore desirable from a therapeutic stand-point.

Regular evacuations from the bowels must be secured for several reasons. In the first place, because the full intestines impede the action of the diaphragm, then because the prolonged retention of fæcal masses in the intestines favors the plethoric condition in which the gut is usually found and which leads to varicosities in the hemorrhoidal plexus, and finally because accumulation of fæces in the cæcum is very apt to produce compression of the ascending vena cava. We need not discuss the unfavorable effects of such compression.

Necessary as it is to secure regular evacuations from the bowels, purgation is inadvisable or even injurious, inasmuch as it may give rise to conditions of weakness, lipothymia or even syncope. It may happen that the patients, who feel weaker as the result of the purgation, state that breathing has become easier, but this relief seems to me to be purchased too dearly. We must here look to the improvement of the patient's nutrition and must administer wine; the meals should be abundant and frequently repeated. The internal administration of iron usually is very beneficial, and the favorable results of the systematic use of waters containing Glauber's salt and, at the same time, a good deal of iron, are thus explained.

Under such treatment a favorable result is often obtained in quite a short time, and careful observation shows that the circulatory conditions have improved with the respiration. The patient informs us concerning the improvement in respiration; the improvement in the circulatory conditions is learned by measurement, which shows that the blood-pressure is increased.

If necessary, atropine or digitalis with and without atropine must be tried in such cases. At all events there is no contra-indication to their use.

Heart failure and hence a disposition to dyspnœa may develop, independent of general obesity, after severe infectious diseases, such as typhoid fever and diphtheria. Another and one of the most important causes of heart failure is over-distention of the heart as the result of strain.

In the last case it seems to be indicated to avoid everything that might produce dyspnœa and to do everything that offers the possibility of improving the lowered heart tonus. For the first reason, absolute rest is indicated; for the latter reason, cardiac tonics should be tried. Among these digitalis occupies the front rank. Da Costa recommended atropine and aconite. I have obtained good results from digitalis combined with belladonna, but have not been in a position hitherto to try atropine alone or in combination with digitalis in such cases.

The treatment of heart failure after typhoid fever and diphtheria and the treatment of the resulting dyspnœa must be directed chiefly to the relief of the general condition of nutrition. Cardiac remedies proper may be dispensed with; we should employ stimulants and tonics, such as alcohol, coffee, iron, if necessary nux vomica.

If dyspnœa is present in mitral insufficiency, with or without stenosis, and if the arterial pressure is also found to be very low, then the question arises with regard to treatment, whether the intensity of the valvular lesion as such or the weakness which attacks a heart suffering from a slight valvular lesion, is to be regarded as the cause of the dyspnœa. A decision is extremely difficult because, as reflection will show, the results of a severe valvular lesion with a sufficient heart muscle may be similar to those observed after slight valvular lesion with insufficient heart muscle.

The first assumption seems to render all treatment useless from the start, so that we must always be guided by the latter assumption. From this standpoint the treatment must follow the principles which I have already laid down with regard to cardiac insufficiency. We must endeavor, by suitable diet, regulation of the secretions and excretions, light exercise (adapted to each individual case), to change the distribution of blood in favor of the arteries and capillaries, and to exercise a favorable influence on the fulness of the heart and, with it, on the nutrition of the organ. Such a change will facilitate, to a certain extent, the escape of blood from the lungs (which is already obstructed by the valvular lesion) and this will improve the expansile or respiratory capacity of the lungs.

Experience teaches that this process is influenced favorably by heart tonics and hence their use appears indicated under certain circumstances. Apart from digitalis with atropine I have seen good results from infusion of adonis (4:150).

It goes without saying that improvement of the heart lesion itself cannot be expected; the most favorable result will be the restitution of the status quo ante.

When a favorable effect is produced, it may be inferred *a posteriori* that the circulatory disturbances resulting from the valvular lesion as such have not been very pronounced. If the treatment is useless, it may be assumed either that the anatomical changes which gave rise to the heart failure had progressed so far that restitution of the function of the muscle was impossible, or the valvular lesion is so pronounced that a change in the muscular action of the heart cannot counteract the injury resulting from the valvular lesion.

Before passing to the treatment of cardiac asthma, I will report a few cases of cardiac dyspnœa from my practice.

IX. CASES OF CARDIAC DYSPNŒA.

I. Mr. E., æt. 51 years; obese for last ten years, respiratory disturbances during past year. Also tendency to palpitation on making an ascent and on mental excitement. Hemorrhoidal hemorrhages. Heart apparently normal in size, sounds clear. May 14th. 1886, pt. weighed 144 kg. Pressure of radial artery 110 mm. Hg. Slight amount of albumin in urine. Treatment: Marienbad cure, exercise, baths, reducing diet. May 21st, weight of body 139 kg. 80 dg., arterial pressure 135. May 28th, weight 135 kg., arterial pressure 145. Respiration much easier, can climb quite well. June 16th, weight 129 kg. 24 dg., arterial pressure 130. Only a trace of albumin found. Striking improvement, which continued during the winter of 1887; during this time the diet was continued and the patient lost 9 kg. in weight. May 23d, 1887, weight 124 kg. 40 dg., arterial pressure 155. Breathing very much improved, no palpitation. Repetition of the cure for prophylactic reasons and in order to effect a further reduction in weight. Diagnosis: beginning insufficiency of the heart and passive congestion of the kidneys. Both relieved by treatment.

II. Mr. B., æt. 55 years. Complains of difficulty of breathing and palpitation, on simply lying down or on movement. Heart sounds normal. Enlargement of the heart not demontrable. June 5th, 1885, arterial pressure 190 mm. Hg., considerable albumin in urine. June 24th, arterial pressure 160; respiration much better, no palpitation, albumin unchanged Diagnosis: arterio-sclerosis, albuminuria. The dyspnœa improves and palpitation disappears, attended with lowering of blood-pressure. Treatment: mineral water cure in Marienbad

III. Mr. M., æt. 65 years. Complains of difficulty in breathing and cough. Examination on June 5th: extensive râles over both lungs, pulse arhythmical; maximum arterial pressure 195, minimum 170. Treament: digitalis with belladonna, in addition to mild mineral water cure. June 21st, arhythmia disappeared, breathing better, production of mucus in the lungs less, only a few râles. Digitalis and belladonna discontinued.   June 26th, arhythmia has reappeared, but less marked; maximum pressure 170, minimum 165; breathing constantly better.   Diagnosis: arterio-sclerosis with corresponding degeneration of the heart.   The arterial pressure diminished, the dyspnœa disappeared, and the stasis catarrh in the lungs improved.   The improvement of the arhythmia was shown by the slight difference between the maximum and minimum of arterial pressure.

IV. Mr. T., æt. 39 years. Complains of palpitation after excitement, also spontaneously in the middle of the night. Dyspnœa on ascending. Patient is an inveterate smoker. Heart normal. June 14th, 1886, arterial pressure 123. Treatment: mild mineral water cure, cold rubbings. June 27th, arterial pressure 132. No palpitation; breathing better. July 2d, patient, who had been doing well, again complained of severe palpitation, which is more frequent at night and is associated with a feeling of anxiety. Arterial pressure 120. It appears that the patient has taken too violent exercise and he is therefore directed to exercise less. July 6th, the patient, who has obeyed orders, is doing better. Arterial pressure 118. July 13th, feels entirely well, arterial pressure 124, palpitation and respiratory disturbances are regarded as the toxic aftereffects of nicotine. The case shows the injurious effect of forced movements. The lowering of the blood-pressure is to be attributed to exhaustion of the heart, perhaps associated with temporary dilatation. The results of the strain disappeared during comparative rest and pari passu with their disappearance the arterial pressure again increased.

V. Mrs. W. æt. 52 years; complains of dyspnœa, also coprostasis with dyspeptic symptoms. Urinary secretion said to be small. Heart's action very arhythmical. Heart sounds clear, heart tender on pressure. Treatment: moderate mineral water cure. July 13th, 1886, maximum arterial pressure 135, minimum 100. Tinct. digit. c. tinct. belladon. āā. July 22d, respiration better, urine more abundant; pressure, maximum 115, minimum 100. July 28th, pulse more uniform, average pressure 120, still arhythmia. Aug. 3d, pulsus bigeminus instead of arhythmia, breathing much better, radial pressure 122. Aug. 9th, radial pressure 120, heart much less sensitive on pressure. Diagnosis: chronic myocarditis (?). Favorable effect of digitalis and belladonna is manifested by abolition of difference between maximum and minimum of pressure; at the same time breathing became easier and the urine more abundant.

VI. Mr. K., æt. 57 years. In 1884 patient had taken a cure at Marienbad for chronic catarrh of stomach and intestines with good effect: reduced his weight 1 kg.; in 1885, repeated the cure. In 1886 he returned but complained more of difficulty in breathing. Also stated that he urinated a larger

amount than before and that the desire to urinate appeared
particularly on walking up-stairs. July 19th, nothing abnormal found in the heart, urine contained small amount of albumin. July 25th, pressure 155, pulse occasionally intermittent,
same condition. July 27th, pressure 160, breathing better.
Aug. 3d, pressure 122 (measured in the morning); auscultation shows reduplication of the first sound. Aug. 10th, patient had great trouble in breathing during the night and
passed large amount of urine. Infus. digital. 0.5–150, tinct.
belladon. 1.0. Aug. 11th, pressure 160, respiration improved.
Aug. 13th, pressure 150, situation unchanged, no dyspnœa.
Aug. 15th, pressure 100, feels weak, but breathing is free.
Aug. 16th, pressure 110, feels better, the intermissions of pulse
have disappeared. Aug. 18th, pressure 140, condition unchanged. Aug. 19th, pressure 145, condition unchanged. The
probable diagnosis appeared to be beginning cirrhosis of the
kidneys. It is noteworthy that the functional disturbance of
the heart was probably aggravated by unusual walking.
This opinion was corroborated by the occurrence of reduplication of the heart sounds and the increased dyspnœa. Digitalis acted favorably; it was followed immediately by temporary increase of pressure, then by considerable diminution
of pressure, and then the pressure returned to its original
height. It is also noteworthy that an increase of the urinary
secretion coincided with increased dyspnœa.

VII. Mr. R., æt. 45 years, complains of difficulty in breathing; moderate degree of obesity, reduplication of systolic
sound. Aug. 21st, pressure 180. Aug. 27th, pressure 170.
Sept. 10th, pressure 160, no reduplication of heart sounds.
Diagnosis: arterio-sclerosis. It is noteworthy that the reduplication disappeared with diminishing pressure.

VIII. Mrs. R., æt. 42 years, marked obesity with dyspnœa.
June 1st, pressure 110. Aug. 20th, pressure 95. Diagnosis:
fatty heart. Breathing improved materially despite the diminution of pressure during the course of treatment.

IX. Mr. H., æt. 40 years, carpenter, complains of great
difficulty in breathing; said to have had left-sided pleurisy
two months before. Heart enlarged toward the right and
left sides. Systole and diastole accompanied by a grating
resonant sound. Dec. 15th, 1886, temporal pressure 100. Dec.
17th, condition unchanged, also complains of feeling of constriction in chest. Temporal pressure 65. Infus. digital. 0.5–
150, sol. atropine (0.3%) 1.0. Dec. 30th, dyspnœa better, only
a diastolic murmur over heart and aorta. Pressure 60. Respiration better. June 8th, 1887, has felt comparatively well
while resting at home. The walk to the Policlinic causes violent dyspnœa with pain in the heart and palpitation. Pressure
70. Jan. 14th, walks better, can stand the walk to the Policlinic.
Pressure 80. Jan. 20th, progressive improvement during com-

parative rest, palpitation and dyspnœa on the slightest work; moderate movement tolerated fairly. Infus. digit. 1-150, sol. atropine (0.3%) 1.0. Feb. 7th, patient begins to do light carpenter work which he tolerates. Feb. 11th, progressive improvement, can work longer and do somewhat heavier work. Feb. 15th, as an experiment the patient receives digitalis alone, without atropine. Mar. 5th, condition unchanged, except that patient states that palpitation occurs more readily during work than while taking the former medicine. Digitalis with atropine is again administered. Mar. 8th, patient states that he can work better than before. Temporal pressure 80. Mar. 19th, patient can work during the morning, but after lunch suffers from gastric disturbance and is apt to get palpitation while working. Pressure 80. Mar. 31st, digitalis discontinued for past 5 days; condition unchanged, pressure 62. April 4th, condition unchanged, adonis with atropine. April 9th, pressure 60, condition unchanged. Thus, from Dec. 17th, 1886, to Feb. 15th, 1887, digitalis with atropine was well tolerated, and progressive though slow improvement occurred after its use. The improvement was especially noticeable from Feb. 5th-7th, when the strong infusion was used. The experiment made between Feb. 15th and Mar. 8th favors the belief that digitalis alone acts less favorably than digitalis with atropine. On the whole, higher pressure was found on the most comfortable days. (The first measurement is not decisive because the patients, as a rule, are excited.) Digitalis was discontinued on account of gastric disturbances and adonis was tried. The arterial pressure then fell, but breathing was not made materially worse. Diagnosis: aortic insufficiency (also pericarditis in the beginning).

X. Mr. B., æt. 38 years, baker. Complains of great difficulty in breathing and palpitation. Heart enlarged in length and breath. Loud diastolic murmur over right heart and aorta. Arhythmia, distinct capillary pulse. Temporal pressure 80. Dec. 20th, treatment: atropine. Dec. 28th, palpitation improved, breathing still difficult. Pressure 92. Arhythmia unchanged. Jan. 20th, palpitation and breathing improved, arhythmia less. Pressure 90. Jan. 27th, condition unchanged, pressure 100. Feb. 19th, exacerbation, severe dyspnœa, cervical veins swollen and pulsating. Pressure 60. Treatment: digitalis 0.5-150 with atropine. Feb. 21st, condition unchanged, pressure 80. Digitalis 1-150 with atropine. Feb. 26th, decided improvement, pressure 87. Mar. 5th, improvement continues, pressure 85. Mar. 19th, material relief, breathing entirely free, pressure 100. Mar. 23d, patient attempts to discontinue the medicine occasionally, but after several days feels the need of resuming it. Diagnosis: aortic insufficiency. It is noteworthy that brief improvement was obtained from atropine and that the exacerbation on Feb.

19th was attended with diminished arterial and increased venous pressure.

IX. Mrs. C., æt. 36 years. Complains of severe dyspnœa, on walking and lying down. Face swollen, also feet. Albumin in urine, which is scanty. Distinct pulsation of jugular vein. Heart's action arhythmical. First heart sound rings like a tense string, cardiac dulness increased to the right. Mar. 7th, temporal pressure 60. Treatment: digitalis with atropine. Mar. 9th, breathing much easier, can lie down, urine more abundant, face no longer swollen, œdema diminishing. Pressure 80. Mar. 13th, improvement continues, œdema disappeared, no albumin in urine. A distinct systolic murmur heard instead of the ringing first sound. Cervical veins no longer distended. Mar. 26th, breathing good, anorexia, digitalis discontinued. April 4th, dypsnœa returns, digitalis resumed. April 12th, no improvement. Temporal pressure 60. Adonis is tried. Diagnosis: mitral insufficiency. Digitalis with atropine had brilliant effects for a short time. A second trial fails. Corresponding with the bad result there was no increase of pressure, which was distinctly noticeable at the first trial.

XII. Mr. D., æt. 44 years, complains of dyspnœa on lying down and is therefore unable to sleep. Diastolic murmur over the aorta, capillary pulse. April 4th, the patient is directed to lie down and the temporal pressure and the boundary between the lungs and liver measured at once. Dyspnœa develops at the end of a minute and the boundary of the lung is found to be pushed downward about 1.5 cm. The arterial pressure had increased from 130 to 170. Treatment: tinct. lobelia with atropine. April 9th, decided improvement, patient can lie down without dyspnœa. April 15th, patient took the medicine until the 12th, felt well until the 14th; then grew worse. Atropine resumed. April 16th, again distinct improvement. April 27th, improvement continues. Diagnosis: aortic insufficiency with high blood-pressure. Atropine with lobelia has good effects.

X. Treatment of Cardiac Asthma.

WE will here discuss chiefly the treatment of the attack itself, because so far as regards the inter-paroxysmal period the same remarks hold good as in cardiac dyspnœa. We must carefully distinguish between the different categories which I have considered in the chapter on diagnosis.

The use of digitalis with atropine is indicated particularly in feeble and, at the same time, irregular heart's action, atropine alone and iodine preparations (potassium iodide or sodium iodide) in arterio-sclerosis. Sodium nitrate and nitroglycerin usually prevent the occurrence of the asthmatic attack, especially when the asthma appears in the train of angina pectoris.

As regards the attack itself, the treatment has been hitherto tentative and by no means assured. Narcotics and stimulants are employed. Among the narcotics morphine is the one chiefly employed, in the form of subcutaneous injections, to abort the attack. Wine, alcohol, ether, camphor and coffee are recommended among the stimulants. There has been hitherto no strict indication for the one or the other, and I will now attempt to discuss the possibility of such an indication.

As regards morphine which, according to numerous statements, may relieve the attack, Traube has said that it acts favorably because it diminishes the irritability of the respiratory centre. A. Fraenkel has also accepted this opinion. If the morphine acted only in this way, its administration would, in my opinion, be strongly contraindicated, because the most important compensatory factor in dyspnœa consists in the activity of the respiratory centre.

The favorable action of morphine may be interpreted, however, in another way. It appears to me to be due to the fact that the drug exerts a material influence on the blood-pressure. Morphine causes lowering of the blood-pressure, as has been shown by experiments (Binz), and, at the same time, the venous pressure falls instead of rising. This would favor its administration in the prodromal stage, and we may assume that its favorable action is obtained chiefly when it is used in prodromal asthma.

So long as the blood-pressure is high and the pulse full and vigorous during the attack, morphine may be administered without fear. It is very possible that early artificial diminution of cardiac tension will prevent the heart from leaving its condition of equilibrium. This would also diminish the arterial tension, but under very unfavorable conditions. In other words, morphine, when administered in prodromal asthma, may possibly prevent the transition into asthma proper.

It is also possible that, in the spasmodic form of asthma which I have assumed, morphine acts favorably by relieving the cardiac spasm.

When we have to deal with the paretic form of asthma, morphine should not be used. According to theoretical considerations, stimulants are then indicated and their action is understood perfectly well. It consists in the stimulation of the depressed heart's action.

Cold must be included among the stimulants. Under its action the tremulous peristaltic movement of the heart yields, as I know by experience, to a regular co-ordinated mode of contraction. Moreover the application of cold to the heart increases the blood-pressure considerably and permanently, as Silva showed.

In addition to narcotics· and stimulants, the inhalation of nitrite of amyl has also been recommended. French writers (Peter, G. Sée) also extol the effects of application of blisters and dry cups.

If there is an abundant secretion of mucus, perhaps associated with œdema, expectorants which may be combined with the stimulants are administered, in accordance with long established custom.

I will now give a tabulated account of a number of cases of cardiac asthma, taken from my practice.

XI. CASES OF CARDIAC ASTHMA.

AGE	SEX	RESPIRATORY SYMPTOMS.	CARDIAC SYMPTOMS.	BLOOD PRESSURE.	REMARKS.
61	F.	Nocturnal attacks of dyspnœa. Feeling of anxiety.	Palpitation during dyspnœa.	8/7 r^1=120 10/7 r=116	Feeling of weakness in both arms during the attack. Increased diuresis after the attack. Marienbad.
49	F.	Diurnal attacks of dyspnœa. Cough and expectoration at times after the attacks.	During the attacks palpitation with feeling of acceleration of pulse and tremor of the heart. Distinct systolic murmur over aorta. Pronounced arteriosclerosis. Heart labile, with tendency to arhythmia.	10/7 r=185 23/7 r=160 28/7 r=140 4/8 r=158	Attacks more frequent in winter. Severe cold causes dyspnœa with cyanosis. Traces of albumin in urine. Arhythmia during transition from higher to lower pressure (July 23d, 30th). Pulse more regular after belladonna. Marienbad.
68	M.	Nocturnal attacks of orthopnœa with cough.	No palpitation. Arteriosclerosis.	r=180 r=160	During the attacks the blood pressure is higher than when the condition has improved. Tinct. lobel. with belladonna acts well. Marienbad. Permanent improvement noted after the lapse of 2 years.
44	M.	Nocturnal attacks of severe dyspnœa, during which râles develop in the chest. Expectoration of bloody sputum immediately after the attack or on the following morning	No palpitation. Heart findings normal during first year of observation. In the second year examination shows prolongation of second sound over aorta and capillary pulse. Insufficiency of the aorta.	1884 1/8 r=185 4/8 r=170 9/8 r=158 17/8 r=150 4/9 r=156 1885 28/7 r=180 4/8 r=165 11/8 r=140 18/8 r=158 22/8 r=150	Albumin in urine. No attacks during course of treatment, during which blood-pressure diminishes. Feels better the following winter. Attacks rare; bloody sputa no longer appear. Milk diet. Marienbad. No medicinal treatment.

1 r signifies the pressure in the radial artery, t that in the temporal artery.

58	M.	Attacks of dyspnœa at night during sleep.	Palpitation during attacks. Arhythmia, distinct pulsus bigeminus in interparoxysmal period.	18/7 $r=150$ 23/7 $r=120$ 26/7 $r=110$ 5/8 $r=130$ 12/8 $r=120$	The heart's action which was at first irregular, gradually improves while the blood pressure is diminishing. No attacks, no medicinal treatment. Marienbad.
36	F.	Diurnal and nocturnal attacks of dyspnœa, lasting a few minutes.	Palpitation after attacks, when breathing has become easy.	9/7 $r=78$ 17/7 $r=110$	Improvement, no attacks, no medicinal treatment. Marienbad.
56	F.	Diurnal and nocturnal attacks of dyspnœa. Distinct emphysema.	Palpitation during attacks.	1882 20/5 $r=165$ 4/6 $r=135$ 1883 29/5 $r=145$ 6/6 $r=130$ 21/6 $r=118$ 27/6 $r=145$ 4/7 $r=150$ 1884 27/5 $r=140$ 30/6 $r=115$	In addition to the asthmatic seizures, attacks of rush of blood to the head with dizziness. Striking improvement after first course of treatment. Marienbad. Improvement continues in following years.
53	M.	Diurnal attacks of dyspnœa after slightest movement. Spontaneous attacks at night. The attacks terminate with cough and expectoration.	Palpitation apt to occur on lying down. Cardiac dulness enlarged to the right. Second pulmonary sound accentuated.	28/6 $r=140$ 16/7 $r=130$	Striking improvement. Marienbad. No medicinal treatment.

CASES OF CARDIAC ASTHMA.—CONTINUED.

AGE.	SEX.	RESPIRATORY SYMPTOMS.	CARDIAC SYMPTOMS.	BLOOD PRESSURE.	REMARKS.
49	F	Nocturnal attacks during sleep. Severe dyspnœa.	Pain in the heart during attacks.	21/6 $r=155$ 31/7 $r=170$	Rush of blood to the head during attacks, face becomes cyanotic and dark patches appear on face. Traces of albumin in urine. The high pressure (170) was observed during severe dyspnœa after rapid walking. Improvement. Albumin disappears. Marienbad. No medicinal treatment.
56	M.	Very severe attacks of dyspnœa lasting ½ hour. Râles in lungs during attack.	No cardiac symptoms.	$r=175$	Cold sweat on forehead during attack, micturition and defecation at end of attack. Improvement in first year (1882). Marienbad. No medicinal treatment. In 1883 and 1884 patient visited Marienbad, but did not consult a physician; died in 1886.
32	M.	Nocturnal attacks of violent dyspnœa.	Emphysema.	$r=148$.	Patient checks attacks by running around room until he perspires. Marienbad. No medicinal treatment. Improvement.
42	M.	Nocturnal attacks after which bloody sputum is expectorated.	Rhythm du galop.	27/5 $r=180$–190 2/6 $r=185$–200 6/6 $r=165$–170 8/7 $r=185$–190	May 25th to June 7th patient continued digitalis which he had taken before. On account of arhythmia, shown by great difference between maximum and minimum of blood-pressure, digitalis is replaced by atropine. Pressure then becomes uniform and arhythmia disappears. No attacks during treatment.

50	F.	Diurnal attacks of dyspnœa with syncope.	Sensation of trembling of heart during attacks.	1/8 $r=130$ 4/8 $r=160$ 15 minutes later 180	Measurement on Aug. 4th made during attack. The already increased pressure quickly rose to 185. Marienbad. No medicinal treatment.
40	F.	Nocturnal attacks of severe dyspnœa, followed by bloody, frothy expectoration.	Aortic insufficiency.	2/7 $r=165$ 8/7 $r=158$	Marienbad. No medicinal treatment.
32	F.	Diurnal attacks of dyspnœa.	Heart dilated on the right; reduplication of systolic sound.	9/8 $r=152$ 11/8 $r=118$	The measurement on Aug. 11th was made during an attack. Unlike other cases, the pressure fell during the attack. No medicinal treatment.
38	F.	Attacks of dyspnœa lasting hours, during which fine and coarse rhonchi develop in chest.	Severe palpitation during attacks, but heart's action does not appear to be increased.	$r=118$	Cold compresses in cardiac region during the seizures have a good effect. Palpitation is relieved and dyspnœa is lessened. Attacks occur during and after menstruation. Marienbad. Cold compresses. Improvement.
49	F.	Attacks of dyspnœa during the day.	Severe palpitation during attacks.	30/7 $r=168$ 12/8 $r=158$	Rush of blood and a feeling as if the blood would shoot suddenly into the head during attacks. In addition to palpitation, sensation of pulsation in neck in carotid region. Marienbad. No medicinal treatment.

CASES OF CARDIAC ASTHMA.—CONTINUED.

AGE	SEX	RESPIRATORY SYMPTOMS.	CARDIAC SYMPTOMS.	BLOOD PRESSURE.	REMARKS.
72	M.	Constant severe dyspnœa; two violent attacks of asthma observed, each lasting 2–3 hours.	Arteriosclerosis.	r =170	Dat … of lungs during … Heart … Stimulants, … dyspnœa. … against the chronic … during …
34	M.	Nocturnal attacks, on waking suddenly from deep sleep.	Palpitation during attacks.	16/7 r=120 10/8 r=126	Marienbad. No medicinal treatment. Improvement.
52	M.	Attacks of orthopnœa at night, lasting hours.	At first visits reduplication of both sounds over left ventricle and slight systolic murmur. Ten days later reduplication disappeared and only the murmur heard.	29/6 r=180 5/7 r=162 8/7 r=180 12/7 r=180	Mild whey cure. Belladonna. Condition unchanged.
52	M.	Attacks of dyspnœa on lying down.	Arhythmia.	20/6 r=165 30/6 r=155 16/7 r=150	Arhythmia disappears in short time, also the attacks. Marienbad. No medicinal treatment. Improvement continues. Fair condition during following winter.
64	M.	Nocturnal attacks of dyspnœa, especially on lying on right side. Attacks in daytime after excitement.	Mitral insufficiency. Diurnal attacks associated with palpitation.	3/7 r=130 8/7 r=120	Tendency to vertigo and dizziness. Marienbad. No medicinal treatment.

57	F.	Nocturnal attacks, lasting several hours.	Aortic insufficiency. Attack begins with pain in cardiac region, then palpitation, then dyspnœa.	17/4 $t=140$ 22/11 $t=135$ 29/11 $t=135$	Policlinic. Atropine acts favorably. Attacks disappear, only palpitation remains. Nitro-glycerin used successfully against latter.
48	F.	Nocturnal attacks.	Mitral insufficiency ; palpitation during attacks.	$t=100$	Policlinic. Atropine relieves the attacks and acts favorably on the heart's action. Improvement continues.
50	M.	Dyspnœa and feeling of anxiety on lying down.	Palpitation, rhythm du galop.	21/4 $t=110$ 23/4 $t=90$	Policlinic. Cannot fall asleep because dyspnœa then develops at once. Tinct. lobel. and atropine. April 23d. dyspnœa disappears during sleep. Improvement continues.
30	M.	Attack of violent dyspnœa, lasting several hours. Attacks in daytime.	Sensation of cardiac spasm during seizures.	14/4 $t=110$	Pallor of face. Abundant expectoration of mucus mixed with blood after attack. Relief from cold compresses. Lobelia and atropine.
42	M.	Nocturnal attacks of asthma, also after eating. Duration 2–3 hours.	Palpitation.	16/3 $t=120$	Atropine alone, nitro-glycerin and sodium iodide without effect. Attacks disappear after digitalis with atropine.

THE

INFLUENCE OF MENSTRUATION

AND OF

PATHOLOGICAL CONDITIONS OF THE UTERUS

ON CUTANEOUS DISEASES

BY

DR. L. GRELLETY,

Consulting Physician at Vichy, Silver Medalist of the Academy, Secretary of
the Therapeutical Society, etc.

INFLUENCE OF MENSTRUATION

PATHOLOGICAL CONDITIONS OF THE UTERUS ON CUTANEOUS DISEASES.

DURING the fifteen years in which I have practised at Vichy, I have frequently been struck by the evident sympathy which exists between the utero-ovarian and tegumentary systems. This is a subject little known and little investigated. It has seemed to me that it would be of some interest to condense within a few pages my personal observations and the notes which I have been able to collect in various authorities.

I shall study at first the influence of menstruation and, after having examined the relation between uterine and cutaneous pathology, I will conclude with certain considerations regarding etiology and therapeutics.

I.

Every one recognizes the coincidence of acne eruptions with puberty and the menopause. Young girls become "pimply," as the common expression runs, when the functions of ovulation are slow in becoming established or are irregular. Similarly circulatory disturbances attend the troublesome period of the fourth decade when menstruation is about to cease. In the interval that local asphyxia, that transient vascular affection, attended by variation in color, occurs much less frequently or it appears to follow delayed menses, uterine troubles, constipation, dyspepsia, and every other affection that may depend on the same constitutional condition. The cheeks

7—8

and region around the mouth are most frequently affected; pustules may predominate, and may cause faces formerly striking to assume an appearance almost repulsive. The public, rarely considerate, knowing that alcoholism prevails in all classes of society, do not fail to suspect the sobriety of such patients, who, on the contrary, often refrain from drinking and eating, or at least take only wine and water and eat lightly, with the quite reasonable hope that they may be able to remedy what they regard as a real infirmity. It is comprehensible that this forms a grave matter for consideration with many women who regard their reputation as highly as they do their health. And they are right, for not only may the ducts of the sebaceous follicles become greatly enlarged, but the subcutaneous connective tissue may share in this enlargement, and may lead to an hypertrophy of the end or alæ of the nose. I published formerly (Gazette Obstétricale, April 20th, 1878) the case of a young lady of twenty-five, who, at almost every menstrual period, had bloating of the face which bore an exact resemblance to erysipelas. I said that it resembled erysipelas, in order to avoid a more exact description; but the term "menstrual erysipelas" has been applied to similar swellings. In his thesis (published April 1st, 1886), M. Tourneux believes that menstruation causes various cutaneous eruptions which serve as a nidus for a supposed streptococcus. In order to explain the periodicity of the erysipelatous eruptions by reproduction, he admits, with Professor Verneuil, the permanence of the microbes of erysipelas at one point on the surface of the body. Hence there is no need of fresh infection at each menstrual period. The patients are auto-infectious; auto-inoculation occurs because the menstrual eruption causes solutions of continuity or excoriating dermatitis. Professor Hardy has applied the term "pemphigus of young girls" (pemphigus virginum) to a bullous eruption which is marked by successive eruptions extending over several months, and which appears only in young girls between fourteen and twenty, in whom menstruation has been interrupted. He has seen only four cases, two which he was unable to follow to their conclusion, and two in which cure resulted from the restoration of the menses.

According to M. Danlos's thesis ("Étude sur la Menstruation au point de vue de son influence sur les maladies cutanées,"

1874) eczema and acne show a preference for the face because of the unusual vascularity of this region.

These eruptions are rare when the periods become established without causing disturbance of the general economy. They usually precede the flow two or three days and fade when the uterine hemorrhage is established. In other cases, adds the distinguished physician of the Tenon hospital, "the menses continue to be suppressed and the eruption persists, as if the hidden trouble from which the system suffered was transferred to the exterior." "In patients with psoriasis, lichen or prurigo, sometimes before the periods the papules become redder and the itching and scratching more marked. However, the effect of the eruption when it occurs is much less appreciable in these dry affections than it is in the case of moist eruptions like eczema and impetigo.

"We have the mildest example of eruptions which develop simultaneously with the menses in herpes labialis, which in many women appears regularly at each period. In most women who are thus affected the herpes is confined to a few patches at the free border of the lips; but, sometimes it is more extensive and the herpetic patches are found also on the cheeks and the nose.

"We may compare with herpes labialis the exacerbation of a chronic pruritus vulvæ, the eruptions of herpes and eczema of the vulva which sometimes occur under the same conditions. Here it is the excessive congestion of the utero-ovarian system which seems to be the cause of the localization.

"In connection with this benign transient affection, let us refer again to the ephelides, following Alibert: . 'The ephelides,' he says, 'are often transient; we observe some which only remain on the skin for a half a day. There are women who are only troubled with ephelides at the approach of menstruation. This mobile characteristic is peculiar to skins that are white and of a very fine texture.' "

M. Danlos admits a third variety of eruptions following the cessation of the menses and appearing after the corresponding periods. This would be a phenomenon comparable to that of menstrual disturbances. To support this statement he simply quotes from Jacquemier: "who has noted in his book on obstetrics the very remarkable fact of fluctuating sanguineous tumors developing periodically on the thighs and in the pelvis. Courty has observed a similar occurrence. M. Potain, in his article on amenorrhœa, after having referred to periodical hemorrhages in women who do not menstruate, adds that the congestion, which in this instance leads to hemorrhage, and which at other times ceases spontaneously, may cause various acute affections, such as erysipelas, urticaria, furuncles, pemphigus, and other cutaneous eruptions, but he makes no mention of the periodic nature of these eruptions."

"M. Hardy considers suppression of the menses as one of the most frequent causes of erythema nodosum. Grisolle expresses the same opinion. Alibert has seen zona develop under the same conditions. It may be asked in this case if this is not a mere coincidence and if it is necessary to see a relation of cause and effect between these eruptions and the absence of the menses. If the periodic character is wanting, it is difficult to decide. If the suppression is temporary, it is conceivable that the development of painful affections, like zona and erythema nodosum, produce a disturbance sufficient to arrest the ovarian menses, and if the suppression is of long duration, it is as simple to refer the absence of the menses to the chloro-anæmia and erythema nodosum to a lymphatic temperament as to make the eruption dependent upon the menstrual suppression.

"This is more readily appreciable when the outbreak of the eruption follows closely the sudden disappearance of the menses. In the following observation, quoted from Alibert, it is impossible to deny this relation: 'A young lady, aged twenty-four, was attacked with a general scaly eruption following suppression of the menses caused by fright. At the end of eight months the uterine functions became re-established and the affection disappeared, not to return.'

"The pruritus vulvæ is above all a complication of the menopause; it is often accompanied by vulvar eczema and intertrigo. In most cases we may refer it to the suppression of the flow, since its onset coincides with the disturbance of menstruation."

"Sometimes," as Franck says, "the bloody secretion is replaced by a muco-lymphatic or by an impetiginous eruption, attended, especially at night, with itching that disturbs slumber and almost defies relief."

In an article, published in the "Concours Médical" for April

14th, 1888, Dr. Deligny mentions various observations on hyperidrosis or profuse sweating, usually confined to a single region of the body, especially the face. He has observed two cases at puberty, though this is peculiar to the menopause. I cannot avoid quoting from this study.

"When profuse sweating," he says, "occurs in certain regions, as the breast, the axillæ, the waist, or the thighs, it often give rise to simple erythema which disappears on slight treatment. Beside the eczema and hyperidrosis, we often observe, at the time of the menopause, the development of eczema in different regions of the body, which appears for the first time, or rather is a recurrence of the same affection which already existed several years before. This is especially noticeable in the case of those suffering from joint affections; we have seen such patients in whom the eczema had presented itself for the first time when the menses were established and the second time at the menopause. The influence of these two physiological revolutions is undoubted.

"Eczema may frequently appear on the ears, or the scalp, the face, or the feet, but eczema genitalium is almost peculiar to the critical period. It begins on the labia majora and extends to the neighboring parts; in one case we observed the eczema occupying the inner sides of the thighs, the perineum, and half of the abdomen.

"This eczema is very annoying by reason of the very intense itching that accompanies it, with evening exacerbations; some patients have attacks that are really terrible. This is not true pruritus, but itching which is no less distressing. It may be added that eczema often succeeds pruritus. Pruritus and the consequent scratching often cause hypertrophy of the pigment at the time of puberty and the menopause. This pigmentation is most frequent on the genitals as a result of idiopathic pruritus, without cutaneous lesions; it is due to marked and oft-repeated hyperæmia of the capillaries. Eczema of the genitals is also frequently followed by temporary pigmentation.

"Rayer, Leroy de Méricourt, Grisolle, and Brière de Boismont have noted peculiar cases of blackish or bluish coloration appearing in cases of sudden establishment of the menopause. Bairé cites a case of Dr. Lyons, of Dublin ('Gazette des Hôpitaux,' 1858), in which the patient was a woman, aged fifty-

seven, whose menses had ceased two years before. She presented a discoloration of the entire skin, most marked on the
hands, toes, and thighs. She soiled her linen and was obliged to
bathe herself more than twenty times a day. Dr. Lyons attributes these phenomena to an excretion of pigment, due to
an effort of nature to continue the elimination from the system. This case of chromidrosis resembles those of Billard,
Bousquet, Neligan, Erasmus Wilson, Hardy, and Leroy de
Méricourt."

Various eruptions then mark the critical period and accom-
pany the flushing, vertigo, and circulatory troubles of every
sort which afflict women between the ages of forty and fifty.
Those who have varices see them enlarge, rupture, and ulcerate. If they tend to stoutness and have soft flesh, pseudo-
lipomata may develop, especially in the neighborhood of the
clavicle. A kind of chronic œdema occurs at this point, with
a collection of lymphoid cells which reproduce. When the
hyperplasia is situated in front of the clavicle, the projection
may be sufficiently prominent to constitute a true deformity
and to necessitate firm compression, to the exclusion of irritating ointments, tincture of iodine, and, above all, surgical
interference.

The influence of the uterus upon the skin is especially manifest during gestation. The pigmentary aberrations then produced have long been familiar; the color and appearance of
the face are greatly changed, and other parts of the body
share in these changes.

Under the name *herpes gestationis* a peculiar eruption has
been described which, according to Duhring, of Philadelphia,
is only the vesicular variety of *dermatitis herpetiformis.*
Toward the fifth or sixth month, pointed condylomata, of the
cauliflower variety and very luxuriant, have been observed to
develop on the vulva and to disappear after delivery. They
may be venereal, but they are not specific or dangerous.

Syphilis itself, when it occurs simultaneously with pregnancy, may assume a very severe form. The flat syphilides,
which must not be confounded with the vegetations above
mentioned, present a papillary hypertrophy such that the tissues have a velvety appearance somewhat as they look under
the microscope. There are several remarkable specimens in
the museum of the hospital Saint-Louis.

II.

If the menstrual function has an action upon the skin, pathological conditions of the uterus exert an influence which is felt in quite another way. I will try to bring out this fact. In his clinical treatise on affections of the uterus (page 104), Martineau devotes a few pages to the study of spots, pigmentation, chromidrosis, herpes, eczema, etc., as resulting from the action of uterine troubles on the skin.

"These changes in the color of the skin which are met with," he says, "in the diseases of the womb and of the mammæ, are not the result of mere chance coincidences; they show that between these organs, physiologically separate, there really exists an affinity, a pathological intimacy.

If we observe that the chloasma persists until long after pregnancy, in fact for several years, we must suspect the presence of a uterine affection following delivery. Amenorrhœa, lactation, and menstrual irregularities have similar consequences, as has been duly established by numerous observations. The amount of pigment increases at each menstrual period, especially in summer.

Uterine affections may produce chloasma as marked as that of pregnancy. Accumulations of pigment at the points of election on the face, the mammary areola, the nymphæ, the linea alba, the anterior aspect of the trunk and the hair sometimes take place during the course of uterine affections in women who have presented none of these during their pregnancies. Long after the menopause (six years, for example) chloasma may appear simultaneously with the development of a tumor, whether ovarian or uterine.

"To the same class of phenomena belongs chromidrosis, which follows menstrual disturbances and uterine irritation. It attends lively emotions and other nervous or nutritive troubles. The close relation of these abnormal stains to uterine disorders is positively proved by treatment; cure the affection of the uterus and the spots will disappear simultaneously.

"In various skin diseases uterine disorders give rise to acute eruptions. Puberty, a period of sexual activity, and the menopause may even, by reason of the changes which they bring about in the system, cause these cutaneous troubles to be dependent upon them. We observe that the first menses are accompanied by hemorrhages and cutaneous eruptions, which improve as the menstruation becomes less profuse and more regular, to suffer exacerbation if menstrual troubles persist. Observations show that when the uterus is imperfectly developed and the menses do not occur, eruptions of an intense and rebellious character appear at the probable time of puberty.

"The fact that herpes coincides with menstruation is a common notion. Courty, Raciborski, Jacquemier, and Potain affirm that the severity of the eruptions is proportioned to the dysmenorrhœa. Professor Potain lays especial stress upon lichen and prurigo. Eczemata and erysipelatous affections are not rare. The absent menses may be replaced by transient periodical eruptions."

Royer-Collard and other writers report cases of psoriasis, eczema, pemphigus, etc., which appear at the same time as the uterine affection and disappear with the latter, to return if the uterus is again diseased. In his "Traité de la Métrite chronique" (translated by Siefferman) Scanzoni affirms that "anæmic women, who have at the same time some affection of the genital organs, very often present various eruptions on the skin, especially when there occurs an intercurrent exacerbation of the uterine trouble. These are chronic eczema, acne disseminata and rosacea, erythematous eruptions, and transient urticariæ, as well as the furuncular diathesis, which is observed most frequently." Hebra also says: "Cases of seborrhœa and alopecia in chlorotic and leucophlegmatic women are due to the same cause as affections of the skin, acne and eczema, that occur in women who are sterile and subject to dysmenorrhœa, that is to a vicious state of the blood." We read in Moritz Kaposi's "Traduction des Maladies de la Peau" (page 377) that in women pruritus is often associated with sexual troubles, dysmenorrhœa, and the menopause. Pruritus of the genitals is often an early prodroma of cancer of the uterus.

Biett and Cazenave have claimed that we should seek for the most common cause of acne rosacea in affections of the stomach, the liver, or the uterus. Hardy affirms, in his "Traité des Maladies de la Peau" (1886, page 533), that these pathological conditions are so frequent without acne that we should only regard them as coincidences; however, he recognizes the fact that pimples on the face occur more frequently in women than in the other sex, that they do not appear before puberty, and that the menopause, as it seemed to him, rather aggravated than produced the affection. Moreover, Hardy says (on page 739) that eczema of the female genitals often arises from a chronic leucorrhœal discharge. A true herpetic vaginitis may thus result, which differs from specific vaginitis in the intensity of the pruritus, the more serious character of the discharge, and the temporary exacerbation which usually accompanies the period of menstruation. On page 598 he admits the simultaneous occurrence of pruritus vulvæ and affections of the uterus and ovaries. "In certain women," he adds, "we observe redness, in fact a true erythematous eruption, extending over the vulva and the adjacent parts; in others we meet with certain superficial excoriations which are apparently eczematous. Pruritus vulvæ, existing independent of dartrous eruptions, venereal diseases, or vaginal discharges, is observed principally at the time of the menopause. Guibout ("Traité des Maladies de la Peau," page 272) affirms that the uterine congestion which precedes and accompanies each menstrual period impresses its marks upon the skin. "You will observe," he adds, "the same chloasma in chronic affections of the uterus, as in the case of fibromata, cancer, and in those profuse and persistent menorrhagiæ, unattended by any organic lesion, which characterize the menopause." As a result of contact with the irritating discharges from the uterus, there has also been observed (rarely, it is true) a leucoplasia with papillary granular projections which resemble the epithelial glossitis that has been roughly designated "psoriasis buccalis."

The prognosis of the lesion dependent upon a uterine trouble is quite grave, since epithelioma may result from it. This mode of termination constitutes an essential difference between it and diabetic eruptions which are associated with sugar in the urine. The latter, on the contrary, are cured by general and local treatment.

Whether chronic herpes of the genitals of menstrual origin is the same as recurrent venereal herpes progenitalis in man or not, it is certain that uterine or vaginal discharges, genital irritation, uncleanliness, and certain occupations (such as the use of the sewing-machine) seem to aid in its development.

The thesis of **F.** Bruneau ("Étude sur les éruptions herpétiques qui se font aux organes génitaux chez la femme" December 18th, 1880) is based on thirty-five cases of herpes genitalis observed at the Lourcine hospital. The author calls attention to the predominance of the eruption on the dependent points. When the cervix uteri was affected, "the posterior lip," he says, "quickly resumes its normal condition, but the anterior may remain ulcerated for a long time. This persistence of the ulceration at this point seems to us to be due to the contact of the stringy, viscous fluid, purulent or not, which escapes from the cervical cavity. The hypersecretion of the endometrium during herpetic eruptions is shown in many of our patients; it has seemed to us in some cases to be due to an extension of the vaginitis, or again, it has seemed as if a chronic leucorrhœa suddenly underwent a temporary exacerbation under the influence of the herpes." Again (page 43) he adds: "As a rule, the utero-ovarian system is not influenced by the discrete herpetic eruption; but it is no less certain that in women who have suffered from some internal trouble, such as ovaritis, metritis, perimetritis, or cervical catarrh, there occurs simultaneously with the cutaneous eruption marked hyperæsthesia of the hypogastric region. Perhaps the discrete herpetic eruption itself which appears on the skin is closely related to the affection of the internal genitals. In nearly all our patients an examination of the cervix revealed a chronic catarrh or ulceration of one of the lips, or else traces of former pelvic peritonitis; the leucorrhœa invariably increased simultaneously with the eruption, without, however, assuming the same profuseness as the uterine discharge which occurs in confluent herpes. How can we explain the phenomena just described? What is the reason of their correlation? What is their point of origin? Whether it is controlled by a general pathological condition or not, this appears to be necessarily dependent on the nervous system. Thus, acne of the face is situated by preference along the expansion of the trifacial which receives filaments from the sympathetic. Besides we are more and more disposed to assign the principal rôle to the nervous system in the production of the various dermopathies."

In his remarkable weekly lessons at the hospital Saint-Louis, Dr. Besnier has affirmed very categorically that sorrow, the troubles of life, and strong emotions exert a certain action on acne, eczema, etc. It is evident that this influence is transmitted through the nervous system.

Dr. Henly has reported, in the "Annales de Dermatologie" (1886, page 350), several cases of psoriasis following fright or different emotions. Leloir has seen a polymorphous bullous erythema in a woman suddenly follow a violent attack of anger ("Des dermatoses par choc moral," 1887). Polymorphous erythema, which appears at certain seasons and especially in women who are debilitated or over-worked, is now regarded as an infectious disease, by auto-infection, not through germs introduced from without. Probably the central nervous system is first affected and the endocardium, especially in the neighborhood of the mitral valve, only undergoes, like the skin, a secondary shock. In the article "erythema" in the "Encyclopædic Dictionary of the Medical Sciences," Dr. Pignot affirms that the appearance of erythema, whether the cause be external or internal, implies more or less the intervention of the nerves that control the circulation in the skin. Nervous action, he adds, is more clearly manifest in the various erythemata which follow visceral lesions. Tooth-rashes in children are evidently of reflex origin. The same is true of the congestive swellings often observed on the face in women when they are the subjects of some utero-ovarian trouble, or even merely at the menstrual period. Moreover, in order to prove that the nervous system is in certain cases the primary, essential, and sole cause of erythematous lesions, he recalls the fact that the various neuralgiæ may cause reflex congestions that are more or less intense and extensive; such, for example, is the redness of the face seen during the painful attacks of trifacial neuralgia.

Purpura, which is not synonymous with hemorrhage, as is generally believed, is in its turn secondary to a disturbance of the vaso-motor centres. The posterior columns of the cord are the intermediate agents. Hence results a local congestion, accompanied by a transudation of the coloring matter of the blood or of a few globules; it is only exceptionally that a hemorrhage is added to this condition.

It is by reflex nervous action that Doctor Leonardi, in his interesting thesis (published January 17th, 1888) explains the appearance of varices in pregnant women. "Supported," he

says, "on this firm and unquestioned basis, the mind, group-
ing all the nervous phenomena which occur during pregnancy,
can assign to their true origin the varices which then appear.
And among the many and varied nervous phenomena of pregnancy, among the psychical troubles (such as longings, per-
versions, and vesaniæ), among the trophic disturbances (such
as chloasma or pigmentation), the different reflex acts (as
vomiting and ptyalism), and the manifestation of nervous and
rheumatic diatheses, varix seems to us to be one of these
phenomena due to the same cause as the others, of frequent
occurrence, and evidently under the neuropathological influence."

In the Dechambre dictionary, under the word "Sympathy," L. Hecht states that "the irritability of the nervous
system explains the frequent occurrence of morbid sympathetic
phenomena in women of nervous temperament and delicate or
enfeebled constitution, especially during the menstrual period;
moreover, the sympathetic nervous phenomena that occur
during the early months of pregnancy may be attributed to a
weakening of the constitution, shown by the diminution in
the number of the red blood-globules, and to the resulting
irritation of the nervous system" (page 678). Again he adds:
"The intensity of the morbid sympathetic phenomena does
not bear any constant and necessary relation to that of the
disease or of the symptoms to which they are due. This intensity may be equal to, or less than the latter. Here, again,
the differences in the degree of irritability of the nervous system may explain the difference in the effects produced."

Moreover, it is rare that the patients, who present at once
a pathological condition of the skin and of the generative
organs, are not extremely nervous. These are most often
women who may be classed under the head of arthritics, or
those who bear an original taint, whose excretory organs act
poorly, and who present great sensitiveness and an imperfect
circulation. I am aware that less importance is now assigned
to diatheses, or so called "cardinal diseases" than in the time
of Bazin. The edifice of arthritis especially has been thrown
down, and we only include under this head gout, with its
chemical peculiarities, and rheumatism, with its special complications. We are more and more inclined to separate arthritis deformans and the whole series of peri-articular pains,

arthropathies, neuralgiæ, etc., which indeed seem to be quite distinct. But, although we pay less attention to former theories and outlines, it is impossible to disregard them entirely, in order to rise above isolated cases and to consider them more generally. As, moreover, therapeutical effects that are apparently the most brilliant are sometimes quite ephemeral, the necessity of discovering and contending with a superior pathogenic cause is imposed upon unbiassed minds.

The practical conclusion to be drawn from these premises is, that, while treating uterine and cutaneous lesions, the entire economy must be acted upon and, as far as possible, the nervous system must be restored to the normal condition of equilibrium. This advice is apparently almost trite, but it is really by no means superfluous, from the fact that each physician tends more and more to confine himself either to a specialty, or to the narrow circle of his own studies. He thus acquires a good competence in some cases, but he is led to neglect other branches of medical science, and above all general ideas; broad conceptions are abandoned, and that too, I do not fear to say, to the detriment of the important interests. What happens? When we find ourselves in the presence of a cutaneons lesion, no matter what, which we have not learned to treat, we do not fail to give the patient an exaggerated feeling of safety, and to encourage his carelessness with the fatal formula: "That will disappear of itself."

Well, it is wrong to hold nature responsible for existing crusts, scales, pustules, comedones, and disease of the sebaceous follicles or their surroundings. We must act, because, unless we do, the evil usually becomes aggravated and makes constant progress. When it heals spontaneously it leaves linear cicatrices, as if from the cut of a pen-knife (by which they are distinguished from the scars of small-pox), after having destroyed the hair-follicle and the sebaceous glands. This is too much. Again, if varicose enlargement continues, bloody operations or scarifications may sometimes be required. Many women, who are obliged by their profession to have unblemished faces, such as actresses, book-keepers, etc., must submit to surgical aid; they might have avoided this extreme measure if they had been treated at the outset.

I shall mention only three therapeutic indications which follow naturally from the foregoing, viz.:

1. Special treatment for the cure of the different forms of metritis and the regulation of the menstrual functions.

2. In general I think that the internal administration of alkalies may be useful; but I shall confine myself to recommending the use of nervous sedatives, above all the valerianates which do not irritate the skin, like bromide of potash, and the removal of all physical or moral causes of excitement. Over-exertion in all its forms, excess of any kind, the abuse of alcoholic liquors, etc., should be on the proscribed list.

3. As regards the cutaneous lesion, the treatment must vary according to the case. It is important for the prestige of the medical profession that it should not be abandoned to the charlatans and quacks of every sort, who pretend to rival in their results the most eminent of the school of Saint-Louis.

TENSION IN SURGICAL PRACTICE

INFLAMMATION OF BONE

AND

CRANIAL AND INTRACRANIAL INJURIES

BY

THOMAS BRYANT, F.R.C.S.
M.CH. (HON.) ROY. UNIV. I.

Vice-President and Member of the Court of Examiners of the Royal College of
Surgeons; Consulting Surgeon to Guy's Hospital; Member of the
Surgical Society of Paris.

TENSION, AS MET WITH IN SUR-
GICAL PRACTICE.

LECTURE I.

ON THE CAUSES, EFFECTS, AND TREATMENT OF TEN-
SION AS MET WITH IN SURGICAL PRACTICE.

WHEN, through the kindness of my colleagues in the Coun-
cil of this College, I was invited to accept the responsible position of Professor of Surgery and Pathology in this honored
Institution, I acceded to their request as a matter of duty,
although with much diffidence, as I felt mistrustful of my
power to bring before an audience, such as is wont to meet in
this theatre, either material of sufficient importance to excite
their interest, or to place it before them in a way sufficiently
attractive to satisfy their critical requirements. To excite
your interest, I have therefore selected a subject with which
practical surgeons have long been familiar, and the importance
of which they have recognized, but concerning which there is
little or no literature—I allude to that of Tension; and should
I fail to make it sufficiently attractive, I have confidence that
it will prove suggestive and tend toward some practical good.
During the last few years the word "tension" has been freely
used by both physicians and surgeons, although it has not
been always employed with the same meaning. In my own
student days it was rarely, if ever, heard; indeed, in a surgical
point of view, it had then but little significance. At the present time, however, we read and hear of it in many senses.
The physician talks to us of arterial and muscular tension,

7—9

and all admit that the word, as thus applied, carries with it deep meaning. The surgeon uses the term as applied to the pressure brought about by the distention or stretching of tissues by cystic or solid growths, by the extravasation of blood, and more particularly, by what is far more common— the effusion of inflammatory fluids. I propose, therefore, in the following lecture, to invite your attention to these different causes of tension, and to trace their effects. I shall do this from the clinical point of view, under the conviction that some practical good may be derived from a full consideration of the subject, and with the hope that some light may thus be thrown upon the diagnosis and treatment of surgical disease.

With respect to the meaning of the word "tension" as employed in surgical work, and particularly in clinical work, it most frequently means the pressure brought about by the stretching or distention of tissue from either the growth of some neoplasm or the effusion of some fluid; tension, in this sense, meaning distention or the stretching of parts by a force acting from within—by centrifugal pressure, as it may be rightly termed. It is, however, applied in another way; that is, to the stretching of tissues which have been divided and brought together by sutures, the strain upon the sutures from the elasticity of tissues being the measure of the tension.

The effects of tension will be found to vary according to the nature of the tissue subjected to its influence. In one of an elastic kind, which yields readily under distention, the effects of tension are neither much felt nor well displayed, unless the expanding or distending force be carried to its full extent; whereas in a tissue which is unyielding and inelastic the mildest distending force is resented, and the effects of tension are forcibly demonstrated. Again, when the distending or stretching medium acts *rapidly*, the tension brought about in the tissues is severe, the symptoms associated with it are serious, and its effects destructive. On the other hand, when the distending, stretching, or straining medium acts *slowly*, tension is seen acting at a lower level, its symptoms are modified in intensity, and its effects qualified. As a general rule, the severity of the effects of tension, as well as the severity of the symptoms which characterize its different degrees, is found to turn upon the acuteness of its action and the elasticity of the tissues implicated. To this rule, however, there are exceptions.

The *ultimate* effects of tension upon any tissue turn, as already stated, upon the elasticity of the tissue and the rapidity with which the tension has been brought about; but they are invariably destructive. Its *immediate* effects, or mode of action, are primarily upon the circulation, particularly the venous; and the pressure from within of necessity tends to bring about—first a slowing of the capillary blood current through the stretched parts, and later on its stagnation, from which the death of tissue follows. When tension is very great, the venous and probably the arterial circulation through the tissues may be absolutely arrested. The nerves of the implicated tissues are at the same time stretched or pressed upon, and as a result pain is produced, and the severity of the pain is determined by the degree of pressure or stretching to which the nerves are subjected, and the character and quality of the nerve supply to the part. The pressure of tension, being centrifugal, acts all round. When the tension has been brought about by the effusion of inflammatory fluids, the effects described are aggravated, for the blood stasis which is well known always to exist in inflamed tissues is encouraged by tension; but of this later on. Where tension occurs in tissues which are not inflamed, inflammation is excited even when the tension is maintained at a low level. Where tension is more severe, destructive inflammatory changes rapidly supervene; but where it is most severe, the death of structure may result from tension without inflammation. Surgeons are familiar with many of these facts in their treatment of wounds; for it is to prevent tension and its evil effects that the drainage of deep, indeed of all, wounds is of such primary importance.

Symptoms of Tension.—The one subjective symptom to which tension gives rise is pain; and this is always found to vary with the degree of tension to which the tissues are exposed, and the quality and quantity of the nerve-supply to the part. Other things being equal, a low degree of tension is associated with slight pain, and a high degree of tension with intense pain. Pain under all circumstances has a common relation to tension. In parts badly supplied with nerves, or at any rate with sensitive nerves, there may be tension and yet no pain, even when from tension the vitality of the stretched

tissues may be destroyed.   An ovarian cyst, for example, may
be so tense as to be deprived of life, and this change be unattended by pain.

The Diagnosis of Tension.—In superficial structures tension can, as a rule, be readily estimated by palpation.   In
deeper parts this may be difficult; in bone, or in the cranial
cavity, it is impossible.   An educated finger can, where palpation is applicable, be brought to diagnose degrees of tension,
as indicated by elasticity and hardness; although where the
tense tissues lie deep this may be difficult.   Where tension is
not acting at its highest force, what is known as fluctuation
may be made out.   Where it is so acting fluctuation may not
be found, only unyielding hardness of the parts implicated.
The degree of tension of the part can, however, be determined
by palpation, as in the eye, when the affected organ is compared with that of the sound side.   The aspect of a tense tissue, moreover, helps diagnosis; its palpable enlargement as
compared with the opposite and unaffected part, and its
stretched appearance, being suggestive.   In such a joint as
the knee this condition can be well observed.   But when the
tense tissue it well covered with soft parts, as in a femur the
seat of periostitis, this observation cannot be made; but even
there the enlargement of the part, and the engorged veins
visible upon its cutaneous surface, are of diagnostic value as
indicative of deep pressure.   The diagnosis of tension of superficial, or comparatively superficial, structures can therefore be
made with accuracy by observation and palpation; whereas,
of deeper structures it can only be rationally inferred.   Its
existence can, nevertheless, be generally tested by surgical
means, and its degrees measured.   I must not, however, allow
myself to dwell upon the diagnosis of tension under all circumstances, but with these general remarks, which have been
made to clear the way, I will pass on to consider the effects of
tension as brought about by the growth of tumors and the
extravasation of blood, to those of tension, the result of inflammation, which probably forms the most important feature
of the whole question.

On Tension from New Growths.—Where tissues are
stretched or distended by a new growth of a non-infiltrating
or innocent character, and its increase is slow, the effects of
tension upon the parts which cover it depend greatly upon

the character of the tissue in which it is placed and its capacity for yielding. Thus, if the tumor be a subcutaneous lipoma, there is rarely pain, as there is no tension; and where pain is present, it is probably due to the implication of some cutaneous nerve. Should the tumor be more deeply placed, as in the breast, which is covered by skin and fascia, and still be innocent, there is not pain of any significance so long as the tumor is small and does not give rise to stretching or distention of its coverings, and what pain exists will probably be of a dull kind. The skin over the tumor, however, as growth continues, changes in appearance, and its normal healthy aspect becomes congested. The engorged vessels are at first few, but later on many, so that at last the surface of the tumor assumes a congested leaden hue. The slow tension of the tissues thus brings about a gradual blood stasis, which passes into or induces the condition of inflammation, and subsequently of ulceration; tension, acting at a low level for a lengthened period of time, always bringing about, although slowly, destructive changes. Should a simple solid or cystic tumor originate in still deeper structures, and be covered with a dense fascia, a very different series of symptoms has to be described. As soon as the fascia becomes stretched or the deep parts distended, tension or centrifugal pressure is produced, and with it pain becomes a symptom of more or less gravity; the character and severity of the pain being determined by the sensibility of the parts involved, the degree of distention of the tissues, and the nature of the nerves involved or pressed upon. For example, a tumor situated between muscles loosely surrounded may, in its early stage, cause little or no pain, since the parts yield under distention; but as it grows and stretches its fascial coverings, pain appears and steadily increases. If growth still continues and the tension of the fascia becomes great, the pain from tension is not only severe, but it is aggravated by the backward or deep pressure of the tumor upon the nerve-trunks of the part in which it lies; the pain of local nerve pressure being added to that due to distention.

Again, should a tumor originate in the sheath of a nerve, pain is at once produced and rapidly increases in severity. The tumor, by its expansile growth not being able to bring about a yielding of the nerve-sheath, presses backward upon the nerve-fibres, and causes suffering. To illustrate these points the following cases may be cited.

CASE I. *Tumor in the Temporal Region beneath the Temporal Fascia and Muscle; intense Local Pain from Tension.* —Mrs. C——, aged thirty, came under my care in January, 1865, for a swelling in her right temporal region, which had been growing slowly for three years. It was hard and fixed to the temporal bone, and pressed forward to the zygoma. The jaw was quite fixed, and could not be moved, apparently because of the stretched temporal muscle. The seat of swelling was the site of intense local pain, evidently due to stretching of the tissues. The lady subsquently died of exhaustion, after nine months of intense suffering.

CASE II. *Tumor in a Nerve-sheath (median); Removal; Cure.*—Miss P——, aged twenty-three, came under my care in August, 1876, with intense pain in the parts supplied by the median nerve of the right hand, contraction of the fingers and inability to extend them on account of pain, and a deeply-seated swelling, about the size of half a hazel-nut, above the anterior annular ligament in the median line of the forearm, The pain had been present for four or five years, but the swelling had only been noticed about six months. It had been mistaken for a ganglion and been punctured, but without relief. I regarded the case as one of neuroma in the median nerve, the tumor pressing upon the nerve exciting pain and forbidding extension. I therefore made a clean cut down upon the nerve, and turned out of its sheath a cystic growth the size of half a nut. (Prep. Guy's Museum, 1614[51]). Immediate relief was given, and a good cure followed, the movements of the hand being perfect.

CASE III.—In 1882 I removed from the upper cord of the left brachial plexus of a lady about fifty years of age a cystic tumor the size of a large hazel-nut, which had been growing for many months. It had caused intense pain down the arm, chiefly in the course of distribution of the musculo-spiral nerve, and from its hardness felt very like an exostosis. On exposure in the subclavian triangle, it was found to be in the upper nerve-cord of the brachial plexus, and within its sheath. On division of the sheath the cystic tumor rapidly enucleated, and this process clearly proved the tension to which the parts had been subjected, and explained the severity of the pain the patient had experienced. Dr. Goodhart reported that the growth seemed to be a blood-cyst. A good result followed the operation, and the lady is now well. (Prep. 1614[5] Guy's Museum.)

When tumors originate in bone, there is, under certain conditions, severe pain, while under others there is but little.

The presence or absence of pain and its degree are regulated by tension. For example, suppose a solid or cystic growth originates in the antrum of the upper jaw. As it grows it tends toward the expansion of its bony casing, and gives rise to tension. As a result pain is induced. This, however, is not often very severe; for the thin bony wall, as a rule, gradually yields to the slow pressure for within, and in due time gives way, thus relieving tension. As a consequence, what pain may have been present, at once becomes ameliorated, and what is left is to be explained rather by the implication of the nerve-trunks of the part than by tension. When the shaft of a long bone becomes the seat of a cystic growth there is more pain, and this pain is from tension, since the wall of bone which surrounds the cyst is dense and unyielding to the centrifugally expanding pressure of the cystic growth. The pain in a case such as this is of the usual aching character, but it does not appear to be aggravated by the warmth of bed, as in inflammatory troubles. These points are well illustrated in the following case.

CASE IV. *Expansion of the Shaft of the Tibia from a Cyst; Trephining of the Bone; Recovery.*—Henry D——, a healthy man, aged twenty-four, came under my care at Guy's Hospital on January 6, 1871, with considerable expansion of the centre of the shaft of the right tibia, which had been coming for two years. He had at times suffered much pain in it, but as a rule it had little more than ached after exertion. He had never had syphilis, and no history of an injury could be obtained. When seen, the bone was found to be expanded in its centre to twice the diameter of the normal bone. The surface of the swelling was much grooved by the cutaneous veins, and the integument over it was slightly œdematous. The parts were tender on firm, but not on gentle, pressure, and the seat of a dull, aching pain, which it is not stated was worse at night. On January 13th I cut down upon the swelling and trephined the bone with a large-sized instrument, and exposed, one inch from the surface of the bone, a cavity as large as a full-sized walnut, which was lined with membrane or granulation tissue, and contained serum more or less blood-stained, but no pus. It was not a hyatid. The bone cut through was denser than natural, and the periosteum over it was thickened. After the operation all pain ceased and a rapid recovery ensued. When I saw the man three years later he was quite well. The enlarged bone had contracted to its normal dimensions, and, beyond the scar of the operation, there were no indications of trouble.

On the other hand, should a solid sarcomatous growth originate in the centre of a dense bone in which there is but little cancellous tissue, such as the lower jaw, in which also there is a canal containing a sensitive nerve, tension in its highest force is the result. This was forcibly illustrated in a case of my colleague Mr. Cock, many years ago at Guy's.

CASE V.—A man had a fibrous tumor growing in the dental canal of the lower jaw, and involving the inferior dental nerve. The agony this man suffered was excruciating, and the relief he experienced by the operation of trephining the bone and removal of the growth was almost magical. In this case the dense bone which surrounded the tumor resisted the effects of steady pressure, and was not absorbed as cancellous bone would have been. The effect of distention or tension upon the walls of the cavity containing the growth was consequently strongly marked and made manifest by pain, which was in its turn intensified by the compressing influence of the fibroma backward upon the dental nerve. As an example of tension brought about by a slowly developing solid growth in unyielding sensitive structures, I am unable to adduce a better.

Tumors of bone do not, however, always distend bone and give rise to tension. Solid sarcomatous growths, which originate in the cancellous tissue of the long bones, rarely do so, at any rate to any extent; for the tumor, as it grows, by its constant pressure steadily causes atrophy or absorption of the bone. And the enlargement of the cavity in the bone going on *pari passu* with the increase of the tumor, neutralizes the effects of tension, and reduces its influence to a low degree. The patient, consequently, under these circumstances, suffers but little, and what pain exists is rarely of a severe or constant kind. As the tumor grows, however, the little pain which may have been present disappears, for the bone after a time becomes perforated by the growth, and tension therefore ceases to exist. With its disappearance pain at once diminishes, and unless the growth presses upon nerves, or structures well supplied with nerves, its progress is probably almost painless. It would appear, therefore, that in the growth of tumors of the soft parts, as well as of bone, the influence of tension is one which cannot be ignored. As the chief cause of pain, directly or indirectly, it is a potent factor, and as a clinical symptom it is one of great diagnostic value.

With this brief reference to tension of tissues, as induced by the growth of solid or cystic tumors, or to what may be called slow tension, I must pass on to consider tension as the result of sudden effusion, and more particularly of blood, to which class the term acute or rapid tension seems applicable. When a cavity or tissue becomes suddenly distended from any cause, the amount of tension which ensues is inversely proportionate to the yielding elasticity of the walls of the cavity or tissue itself. The effects of the distention turn upon the degree of tension that is produced; and the symptoms to which the tension gives rise vary with the nerve supply to the part. Thus, in every-day practice, where blood is effused, as a consequence of an injury, into subcutaneous tissue which is thin, elastic, and capable of distention, as in the eyelids and scrotum, the patient experiences but little pain or other morbid sensation beyond a feeling of fulness, unless the hæmorrhage is great and the parts are stretched to their utmost. Whereas, should the effused blood be rapidly poured out into the skin of the ear, the junction of the nose with the upper lip, parotid region, or outer labium, parts which are not only sensitive but incapable of much stretching, the pain is severe, and this symptom is entirely due to the stretching or tension of the tissues into or beneath which the blood has been extravasated. Where no distention of parts exists, and as a consequence there is no tension, subcutaneous hæmorrhage may take place to a considerable extent and give rise to little local pain or other symptom than local swelling. The pain which attends subcutaneous hæmorrhage is in proportion to the degree of stretching or tension of the parts implicated. No tension means little pain; severe tension severe pain. When hæmorrhage takes place beneath the deep fascia which binds down tissues, pain is often severe; the distention of the fascia, the tension of its fibres, and the centrifugal pressure generally, being its cause. This is fairly illustrated in a case of simple fracture above the ankle, and in most sprains of joints attended with blood effusion. As the blood is absorbed, pain goes and repair progresses.

When we consider the subject of hæmorrhage into cavities, and the symptoms it produces, the same conclusions are arrived at. Thus, a patient may bleed to death from hæmorrhage into the peritoneal cavity, without manifesting any other symptoms than those which are described as general. There is no pain. The same may be said with respect to bleeding into the thorax. In neither of these cavities can tension, as a result of bleeding, be well produced, and as a consequence there is no pain. In intracranial hæmorrhage, where there is no yielding of external tissues, but only backward pressure, the effects of tension are very marked and destructive.

When bleeding, however, occurs into cavities which are within the range of distention, and in which, therefore, the effects of tension or centrifugal pressure may be felt or demonstrated, a different result has to be told. Thus, when a knee-joint is the seat of fracture of any of its bones, and as a consequence hæmorrhage takes place into the joint, the cavity may become so distended with blood, and thus tense, as to produce severe local pain and general disturbance, which, if not relieved, may be followed by the destruction of the joint. The eyeball may be the seat of extravasation of blood into its anterior, middle, or deeper chamber, and its presence be unattended by any pain, unless the hæmorrhage be sufficiently extensive to distend the globe and give rise to tension. The tunica vaginalis of the scrotum may likewise become the seat of hæmatocele, and the amount of pain associated with it will turn upon the rapidity of the effusion and the mechanical distention or tension of the walls of the cavity into which the blood has been poured. The pain in all these cases, when it occurs, is clearly dependent upon tension.

When hæmorrhage takes place into deep, unyielding, and possibly sensitive structures, the degree of pain to which it gives rise can hardly be measured.

CASE VI.—Some twelve years ago I was asked by the late Dr. Remington, of Brixton, to see a fine young man, of about twenty-five, who, the day previously to my visit, had received a blow upon one of his testicles, and from the time of its receipt had suffered intense local pain, which opiates and local treatment had failed to relieve. When I went into his room the patient was walking about with his hands grasping his genital organs, and moaning with agony. In one testicle there was intense pain of a throbbing character, and the pain had since the accident been so severe that the patient said he had neither slept nor rested. I examined the scrotum, and failed to see any external signs of injury. The painful testicle was, however, larger than its fellow, and this enlargement was in the body of the gland. On careful manipulation, I made out a tense point in the body of the testis, and this point was painful. The man's temperature was normal, and there did not appear to be any local heat about the testicle. I came to the conclusion, therefore, that in this case the patient was probably suffering from hæmorrhage into the body of the testicle itself, and that the intense pain which was experienced was due to tension. I consequently persuaded him to allow me to introduce a fine exploring trocar and cannula into the swelling; which I did, giving exit to a jet of blood or blood-stained serum which spurted out in every direction. With this spurt all pain ceased, and a rapid convalescence followed. That the pain in this case was due to the tension caused by the rapid effusion of blood into a sensitive gland encased in an unyielding fibrous covering—the tunic albuginea—there can be little doubt; and with the diagnosis the treatment was simple.

CASE VII. *Puncture of the Testicle in the Operation of Tapping a Vaginal Hydrocele; Hæmorrhage into the Testicle Producing Pain from Tension; Operation and Recovery.*—Mr. D——, aged twenty-one, consulted me in March, 1871, on the advice of Dr. Tyson, of Folkestone, for some affection of his left testicle, which had been swollen for ten years or more, but had only been painful since it had been surgically treated. One month before I saw him he went to a surgeon,who tapped the swelling and drew off a blood-stained fluid mixed with blood-clot. When the instrument was withdrawn the swelling steadily reappeared, and the testicle became the seat of intense pain, the pain passing up the cord. Since then the swelling had steadily increased, and the pain had been sickening. When I saw him the testicle was the size of a cocoanut, ovoid in shape, smooth, and very painful. It was not hot. Thinking the case might have been a hæmatocele of the tunica vaginalis, although the extreme pain suggested something else, I at once explored the tumor by means of an incision, and found that it was a hæmatocele—but of the body of the testicle, and not of the tunica vaginalis. There had evidently originally been a hydrocele of the tunica vaginalis, for when I operated there was evidence of this fact; but the testis itself had been converted into one large cyst containing broken-up and fœtid blood. I removed the whole organ, which was useless, and a good recovery ensued. In this case the testicle had doubtless been punctured when the hydrocele was tapped, and as a consequence hæmorrhage followed the puncture. The pain which came on after the operation of tapping, and which had not existed before, was clearly due to tension within the testicle brought about by the bleeding.

I have another case of tension brought about by the extravasation of blood, which I should like to relate, since it is well in point.

CASE VIII.—In 1877 I saw with Dr. Donald Hood, of Green Street, but then of Caterham, a gentleman who in a hunting accident had ruptured his urethra, and was suffering from retention and urinary extravasation. These symptoms were relieved by perineal incisions and catheterism, and all went well for three days, when bleeding from the urethra again appeared, associated with agonizing pain at the root of the penis. On examining him through the wound, which I then did, I found the bulbous portion of the urethra very tense and exquisitely painful, and it was clear that this tension of the part was due to fluid. I accordingly made an incision into the bulb, and with the incision what must be described as an explosion at once occurred, for blood was scattered in all directions. Copious bleeding followed, which clearly came from the artery of the bulb. The hæmorrhage was controlled and all eventually went well. The tension of the bulb in this case from arterial hæmorrhage was testified by the presence of intense local pain, and it was proved by the explosive sound caused by the division of the distended tissues, as well as by the scattering of blood upon the operator and his assistants as soon as the retaining capsule was divided.

Tension in these cases was acting at its highest force, and, as the parts implicated were highly sensitive, severe pain was the result. Tension being relieved in every case, pain was banished, and repair went on in its normal way.

This accumulative evidence which I have brought together, I think, therefore, points to one conclusion—that tension and pain as met with in cases of growths, expanding tissues, or of hæmorrhage into tissues and cavities, are closely related; in fact, that pain in these cases is the result of tension.

On Tension the Result of Inflammation.—I will now pass on to consider the subject of tension in its relation to inflammation, and need hardly remind you that swelling is one of the classical symptoms of the process, and that this swelling is due to the exudation from the slowly flowing blood stream of corpuscular liquid which passes through the inflamed tissues, and which may lead up to blood stasis; this slowing of the blood current and consequential exudation forming Sanderson's central phenomenon of inflammation. Indeed, these elementary truths are such as every student and practitioner should ever have before him when considering any inflammatory affection, for they form the key to an intelligent appreciation of the local symptoms and pathological phenomena of every case. When effusion takes place, therefore, into any tissue which is inflamed, swelling follows, and the amount of swelling turns upon the character of the tissue into which it takes place. Where there is much connective tissue, and the parts are elastic and yield to distensile forces, the swelling is great; but as the resistance to it is not serious there is little or no tension; such an effect only follows extreme distention. Where the effusion is poured out into connective tissue contained in fibrous sheaths, or beneath or within fascial envelopes, as in joints, the distending force is great, and tension consequently is often found acting to a high degree; and where it exists in bone or in unyielding bony cavities, tension of the severest type is met with.

That local pain is a sign of tension all agree, although all will probably not consent to the opinion that tension is the cause of most pain. In inflammation, however, I think there can be little doubt as to the truth of this view, for pain and tension seem to be practically proportionate, the former being felt in exact proportion to the degree of the latter, and rising and falling with its force. Indeed, in a clinical point of view, I believe that the pain of tension should be regarded as a test symptom of inflammation. Where there is feeble tension in any inflamed part, the pain hardly exceeds that of uneasiness; where there is high tension, the suffering is severe; where tension is relieved by natural or surgical processes, pain goes. Under all circumstances, the presence of pain in any local inflammation may be accepted as a sign and indication of tension and a call for its relief. When pain is increased at night —that is, when the patient is warm in bed and the circulation is acting at its highest force—the probabilities are that the affection is inflammatory, and that such increase in the force of the circulation which is promoted by warmth tends toward the production of tension or its aggravation.

The *effects of tension* upon the inflamed tissues depend much upon its degree. When it is but slight, tension may tend only toward the maintenance of the inflammatory process; when it is more severe, it must help, not only to keep up, but also to aggravate, the action; and when it is acting at its highest force, there is no escape from the conclusion that it assists powerfully to bring about the destruction of the tissues which feel its immediate influence, and to encourage inflammatory action in such as are more remote. How it helps to bring about destruction of inflamed tissue is not difficult to understand, since it acts in tissues that are inflamed in the same way as it has been shown to act in such as are not so affected—that is, by helping to bring about blood stasis. In tissues that are inflamed the tendency to blood stasis invariably exists, so, with tension acting upon them, there can be no surprise that this blood stasis, with all its evils, is greatly encouraged. To say, as students are taught, that death of inflamed tissue from tension is due to the cutting off of blood supply to the inflamed part is a fundamental error. The blood is in the tissues, but it is stagnant and not circulating. The death of inflamed tissues from tension takes place, as it does in a strangulated part, from the stasis of its own venous blood. It is a form of static, not of anæmic, gangrene—of death of tissue brought about by the stagnation of the blood in the capillaries, and not by a want of blood supply.

I will now proceed to illustrate the effects of tension upon different tissues; and first of all let me take as an example a case of cutaneous erysipelas, and assume that it has attacked the skin of a part loosely connected with the deep tissues and capable of ready distention. The local sensation produced by the disease does not go beyond a sensation of stiffness—it does not amount to pain; but let the inflammation spread to parts so placed as to be anatomically capable of but little, if any, distention, how different then are the symptoms complained of, and how soon inconvenience passes into pain, even of an acute kind. Let any one who has had erysipelas, or any inflammation of the nose, upper lip, nape of neck, or ears, answer this question, and at the same time tell us the comfort he experienced when the tension was mechanically relieved. In this example of cutaneous inflammation the view that local pain is fairly due to tension is well supported, and the relief that is given to the symptoms by local treatment helps the conclusion.

Let me now draw an illustration of the effects of tension from inflammation of a deep structure bound down by inelastic tissues, such as is met with in a familiar example of thecal inflammation. What pain is at once experienced here from the first onset of the trouble, and how rapidly it intensifies!

What destruction of tissue follows if relief be not given! And what comfort and rapid recovery ensue if the case be rightly treated! These facts are familiar to us all, and yet I am rash enough to say, even in your presence, that I am somewhat in doubt as to whether the generality of surgical practitioners realize their full meaning, and so conform their treatment to the exigencies of the case as to give their patient the best chance of a recovery. Let me take this example of thecal inflammation, therefore, as a text, and enlarge upon it, first of all following its natural course. Inflammation attacks the tissue; the capillaries of the inflamed part consequently become more or less thrombosed, and as a result effusion takes place. The effusion is confined in a tight channel, the walls of which are but feebly capable of yielding, and as a consequence the fluid, pressing centrifugally everywhere, not only violently stretches or distends the tissues in which it is confined and gives rise to high tension, but also seeks a vent by flowing in the line of the least resistance along the course of the tendon up the fore-arm. From this pressure, if relief be not given, death of tissues speedily follows, this result being brought about, as already described, by the influence of tension in encouraging the blood stasis which forms part of the process of inflammation. With the death of tissue suppuration within the thecal channel takes place, rupture of the weakened thecal structure follows, and in the end comes the external discharge of the dead tissues, with probably many burrowing abscesses. A vast amount of destruction of tissue from tension has taken place quite unnecessarily, since by active and scientific early treatment a very different result could have been obtained. The cause of all this extensive trouble was practically due to tension, and if this had been relieved in its early origin recovery would have been possible, nay probable, without loss of structure.

The inference to be drawn from such a case as this, and from all others like it, is that to relieve tension by giving vent to pent-up fluids in distended tissues is a primary surgical duty, and that this practice cannot be applied too early, may safely be dogmatically advised. At the present day among experienced surgeons it may be said that this practice is fairly universal; but is it? Is there not even now a lingering dread in some surgeons' minds of incising or even deeply puncturing an inflamed tissue before suppuration has commenced? And have not many of us heard, when an incision has been made into such inflamed tissues as those just mentioned, something like an observation of pleasure that a fluid like pus has been seen to flow, as if to justify the act? Whereas the surgeon's pleasure should be where his duty lies, to give vent to pent-up inflammatory fluids before suppuration or other destructive changes have taken place. In my own practice, I as a matter of routine cut down freely and immediately upon a finger the seat of thecal inflammation, and always congratulate myself that I have done so when only serum and blood escape, and no pus; for the existence of pus means destruction of tissue under most if not all circumstances, a result which should be avoided.

Again, let me give another example. A joint, let me say a knee- or hip-joint, becomes inflamed and acutely distended with inflammatory fluids. The synovial membrane as a consequence becomes tense from distention, and there arises the natural fear that disorganizing changes in the joint will soon occur, if the tension thus produced be not relieved. The joint consequently is either aspirated or punctured with a tenotomy knife through a valvular subcutaneous wound, to relieve tension, and *some little* of the serous exudation is drawn off or allowed to escape into the connective tissue, where it will become absorbed. This little operation at once not only relieves pain by relieving tension, but it does more, for in a few days the fluid which was left in the joint disappears by natural processes, and convalescence is soon established.

An acutely inflamed bursa may be similarly dealt with, and an equally good result expected; and in the following case a like treatment of a hydrocele was followed by a like result. The case I give in the words of Dr. Bower Harrison, of Manchester.

CASE IX.—"In March, 1878, I was myself the subject of hydrocele of about seven or eight months' duration. On the 20th instant, on getting out of a warm bath, I introduced an ordinary hypodermic syringe into the hydrocele, and, using it as an aspirator, removed about ten minims of fluid. A few drops of water remained on the spot where the syringe had been used. This dew continued to show itself for some time afterward, while a perceptible softening of the whole tumor took place. In a few days the hydrocele had perceptibly diminished, and in a short time had wholly disappeared. It never recurred. In mentioning the case to my friend, Professor Lund, of Manchester, he expressed himself as much interested, saying that he felt convinced that the diminution of tension in the case of an imprisoned fluid greatly promoted its absorption. He further stated that he was in the habit of speaking of this to his class as an important *law.*" I am quite convinced that our friend, Mr. Lund, is right in this matter. Indeed, I have for years taught this law myself. The withdrawal of some of the distending fluid from a tense synovial or serous sac not only relieves pain with the tension of the part, but at the same time frees the lymphatic, venous, and arterial circulation from the impeding effects of local pressure, and thus, by encouraging a more normal or healthy action of the vessels generally, tends toward the relief of the blood stasis, which is the main important pathological condition of inflammation, and thus helps toward recovery. In the same way the contents of an abscess may often become absorbed by natural processes, after a sufficient quantity of its contents has been withdrawn to relieve tension.

Again, glaucoma attacks the eyeball of a patient, and, whether acute or chronic, is attended by distention of the globe of the eye and extreme pain, the result of tension. Its treatment consists in an operation for the relief of tension, and without an operation in one of its forms recovery is considered by all authorities to be hopeless. "We must always bear in mind," writes my colleague Mr. Higgens, "that an operation to be successful must be performed early," the author meaning by "early" that it should be undertaken before the secondary changes in the structure of the eye, the result of distention, have been brought about. Surely this principle of practice, which is so binding and valuable in the treatment of an affection of the eye due entirely to tension, should be equally binding, as it would be equally valuable, in the treatment of all local inflammations in which tension has such a pervading influence.

Acute inflammation of the pulp of a tooth affords another illustration of the evil effects of pent-up inflammatory fluids upon surrounding parts, and of the severity of the local symptoms which must be attributed to such a cause. "In this case," writes Moon, "every factor for the production of agonizing pain is present; the distensible pulp, largely supplied with nerves, undergoes vascular engorgement within an unyielding ease—closed in all parts except at the aperture of

exposure." The trouble, if left unrelieved, soon ends in the
death of the plup, and too often in the extension of the inflammation to the periosteum of the jaw-bone and surrounding
parts, with its ultimate bad effects. How many of these consequences may be avoided by judicious treatment I must not
now stop to inquire; clearly the majority. Where the antrum
of Highmore is involved in acute inflammatory trouble the
same conditions are present. Tension, and as a result, pain,
are prominent symptoms, and these are only to be relieved by
surgical action.

In the surgical affections of the ear many illustrations of
the same truths may be found. In furuncles and inflammation
of the external meatus, as is well known, severe pain is experienced, the pain being the direct result of the unyielding
condition of the skin and connective tissue in which the inflammatory process originates, and the effects of the tension
being indicated by the throbbing pain, the feeling of fulness
in the part, and the general febrile disturbance which in these
cases is so often present. In acute inflammation of the middle
ear, or in the acute grafted upon a chronic affection, the evil
effects of tension are forcibly illustrated, for in such cases the
walls of the inflamed cavity are chiefly bony; and where this
is not the case, the foramina, which communicate, on the one
hand, directly externally, and, on the other, indirectly internally, with the cranial cavity itself, are only covered with
a membrane. When this cavity, therefore, is filled with inflammatory fluid, and the inflammatory process continues, the
full effects of the centrifugal distending force upon the walls
of the cavity, in bringing about tension on its yielding and unyielding walls, is very marked. Indeed, it may be said without fear of contradiction that there are few local inflammatory
affections which give rise to more severe local or general
symptoms than otitis media. The severe and agonizing local
pain, radiating in all directions, the high fever and general
constitutional disturbance, and too often the brain symptoms
and complications which mark its natural progress, all point
to the evil effects of pent-up inflammatory fluids, while the
rapid influence of sound local treatment support a like conclusion.

Again, in inflammation and suppuration of the kidney
brought about by the presence of a calculus or any obstructive

cause in the urinary track, the same conclusions find full support. In these cases the lumbar or kidney pain—usually synonymous—turns almost entirely upon the tension or distention of the pelvis of the kidney. When, from any cause, the ureter of a kidney thus affected is obstructed, pain is caused or increased; when the ureter opens and allows the free exit of pus, pain diminishes, or even disappears. The disappearance of the pain depends entirely upon the unblocking of the ureter and the consequent relief to tension of the pelvis of the kidney. On this account a patient with a disorganized kidney may go on for years, suffering when obstruction to the flow of pus takes place, and being comparatively easy between whiles.

Indeed, in any suppurating cavity the same cause and effect can be traced. Retained pus always gives rise to pain more or less severe, and its severity turns upon the distention of the abscess cavity. When the tension is brought about suddenly, and is severe, the pain is great, as in acute abscess; where it is produced by a chronic process, the pain often is but little, tension being little. The pain of abscess generally turns almost entirely upon the tension of the walls of its cavity, and its severity upon the rapidity with which the tension is brought about, the anatomical surroundings of the part having its due influence. If further illustrations of the effects of tension were needed, abundance might be adduced from the surgery of inflamed periosteum and bones. For my present purposes such are not required, although in another lecture I propose to bring the subject before you as a whole.

I must, however, as a final and possibly convincing exemplification of the truth of all my preceding remarks, refer to *tension as seen in wounds,* the result of either accident or operation.

In the treatment of wounds, and more particularly of deep wounds, the evil effect of tension upon the process of repair is well recognized; and it may, I think, be said that, if wounds are treated upon approved modern methods, the subject of the wound be healthy, his surroundings wholesome, and due provision be made against the possibility of any fluid exudation from the wound being retained, so as to give rise to tension, the surgeon may with confidence look forward to the reparative process being carried out without the slightest trace of inflammation, and without pain; whereas, if this important point of treatment be forgotten, disregarded, or inadequately provided for, the slightest trace of tension upon the margins of the wounds, or of distention of its depths, will to a certainty show its evil effects, not only by preventing quick or any form of union, but also by changing the quiet physiological process of repair into the pathological which we call inflammatory, and thus set up a destructive in the place of a constructive process.   This result ensues quite irrespective of the form of wound dressing that may have been employed.

I should like from this chair to repeat what I have been long teaching, and what modern surgery has done so much to inculcate, that repair and inflammation are not only not identical but incompatible; that repair is a physiological constructive restorative process, while inflammation is a pathological destructive one.

When inflammation attacks a wound that is healing by John Hunter's first intention, arrest of repair first appears, then disrepair, and the injured tissues will, when the inflammatory process has subsided, have to heal by granulation. Should, by some chance, inflammation attack a healthy granulating surface the granulations will at once break down, and the molecular death of tissue, or the ulcerating process, take the place of what had been the reparative; the constructive process in both cases having been destroyed by the inflammatory and exchanged for the destructive.   In the repair of all parts which have been damaged by the inflammatory process, inflammation must cease before repair begins.   I would that this view of repair and inflammation were more generally entertained; it would help clinical surgery, for it would lead all surgeons, in their treatment of wounds, to avoid and guard against every outside influence that can possibly give rise to the over-action which we call inflammation, whether such be the introduction or germination of microbes from without, or the effects of tension from within.

I am not, however, here discussing the general causes of local inflammation.   My object is simply to show that tension in wounds may either originate or keep it up; where the tension is severe, acute inflammation will follow, as in tissues which are not wounded; where it is acting at a lower level, it will still be destructive, although less so in degree. Should sutures of any kind be introduced to keep the edges of a wound together, and upon one or two the effects of tension be felt, at such points local inflammation will originate and pass on to ulceration. Whereas about the other sutures at which there is no tension, and yet which in other respects are similarly placed, no such action will be found to exist. And this result will occur quite irrespective of the nature of the sutures employed, and however carefully the antiseptic or other treatment of the wound be carried out. The local inflammation in these cases is clearly due to local causes, and to no other.

Again, if in a deep wound, blood or serum is allowed to collect in sufficient quantities to separate its adjacent surfaces, and by so doing give rise to tension of the surrounding tissues, inflammation will to a certainty follow, and such will pass on to suppuration if the tension be maintained. Whereas, if the tension be relieved soon after its appearance, the inflammation will soon subside, and the reparative process resume its physiological work. The wounded surfaces, however, under both cir-cumstances, are not likely to unite by quick or primary union, but by the slower process of granulation. In fact, the influence of tension upon the repair of wounds, both as a cause of inflammation as well as a source of its persistency, supports, if it does not prove, the following conclusions which the consideration of tension associated with other conditions has led me to draw.

1. That tension has a wide pervading influence in clinical surgery, as well as a decidedly marked effect upon the progress of disease.

2. That it is the product of many causes, and that these, for clinical purposes, may be conveniently divided into the inflammatory and non-inflammatory.

3. That it stands foremost among the causes of pain, and in inflammatory affections it is probably the chief pain factor.

4. That where the causes are not inflammatory the tension to which they give rise will, if maintained for any time at a low level, or rapidly rising to a high level, excite inflammation in the tissues affected.

5. That, where the cause is inflammation, the tendency of tension is to keep up or intensify the inflammatory action, and strongly to encourage its destructive influences.

6. That tension in every degree has a destructive tendency, and the rapidity of the destructive process has a direct relation to the acuteness of the tension.

7. That, as in wounds the slightest degree of tension is injurious, so, in their treatment, the use of the drainage-tube, or due provision for complete drainage, is a point of such primary importance as to relegate to a secondary position the mode and character of the dressing which is employed, since a want of attention to the efficient drainage of a wound under every form of dressing is followed by the same result.

If these conclusions be true, and I am satisfied that in the main they are, two others ask for expression, the first being the value of local pain as a clinical sign of tension and an indication for local treatment; and the second the expediency, if not necessity, of relieving tension as speedily as possible under all circumstances. To both of these points I must briefly call your attention.

The Treatment of Tension.—If arguments were needed to support the view that the pain associated with a local inflammation is chiefly due to tension, they would be found in its treatment; for if the local inflammation be situated in an extremity—say a hand—the local pain will at once be relieved by such a simple measure as elevation of the limb; the elevation tending at once to empty the venous capillaries, and at the same time to diminish the force of the arterial blood supply to the inflamed parts, and thus to relieve the blood stasis and the tension resulting from it. On the same principle, the arrest of the flow of blood through the main artery of the limb by temporary pressure, or the more or less complete and permanent occlusion of its lumen by temporary or permanent ligatures, has been found to act beneficially. By such means pain is at once relieved, and other advantages at the same time secured. Local venesection, leeching or cupping in either of its forms, must also act in the same way, by relieving tension; the local abstraction of blood from the seat of an inflammation or its neighborhood so emptying the congested vessels in the outer zone of an inflammatory centre as to encourage the circulation of the part generally, and by so doing give relief to the overgorged and dilated capillaries of the centrally inflamed tissues. The local loss of blood, even when very limited in extent, relieves tension, and with it its diagnostic symptom, pain. In the same way, it is probable that cupping, dry or moist, and counter-irritation, have a beneficial tendency, and that these means, by drawing blood to a part not too remote from the seat of inflammation, help to relieve the congested capillaries in the focus of disease, and thus to favor the circulation through them; this favoring of the circulation tending, of necessity, to discourage blood stasis and hyperæmia, to relieve pain, and to help the natural powers to bring about a cure of local inflammation by resolution.

In the inflammation of soft parts, where the stretched tissues are elastic, their natural resiliency may have a beneficial influence toward the re-establishment of the circulation and the favoring of a recovery by resolution; whereas, in the inflammation of the more inelastic and unyielding structures such as the eyeball, middle ear, joint capsules, periosteum, and bone, no such help can be counted upon; for when these parts become the subject of acute or chronic inflammation, and consequently the seat of tension, such tension and inflammation, unless relieved by surgical art, will continue, and thereby bring about permanent or destructive changes in the inflamed parts, the result being in one case thickening and consolidation of structure, and in the other suppuration, ulceration, or death of tissue. It would therefore appear that in the treatment of local inflammation the relief of tension is an all-important point of practice to be followed, and that the means which in any individual case can best fulfil this object will be the right ones to adopt. In some cases the relief may be brought about or helped by position, in others by pressure. In acute cases it is only to be efficiently produced by a puncture, incision, drill, or trephine into the tense tissues or cavities; whereas, when the soft and elastic structures of the body are the seat of trouble, local venesection, cupping, or the application of leeches may suffice and it would be well if such means were more frequently employed. But wherever tension may be found, and in whatever tissue it may be situated, means must be employed for its relief; since, so long as it exists, the causes which led to it will probably continue, unless by the natural progress of the case tension becomes relieved by the destruction of the structures which are under its influence, or natural processes are sufficient to bring about a cure.

Where pain is present as an indication of the existence of

inflammatory tension, the surgeon has a guide of great value to help him to the right treatment of his case, and it is one which he should rightly use; although where pain is absent or but feebly expressed, there is the same necessity to relieve tension where it exists, for tension may be present even with distention without giving rise to pain; as, for example, in certain forms of peritoneal inflammation. In these cases, however, the same line of treatment is called for, and the same principle of practice is applicable as in others to which attention has been drawn; for, with an abdomen full of fluid, which is pressing in all directions upon veins, lymphatics, arteries, and viscera, with an embarrassed circulation, and an arrest of all physiological action of the organs implicated, how can any curative action be expected to take place? Let the distended abdominal cavity be relieved by the evacuation of its contents; let some or all of the inflammatory products which may retard repair be washed away and the circulation be disembarrassed; let the viscera be freed from all pressure, and the physiological action of all these important parts be allowed to have fair play, and then recovery may be brought within the bounds of possibility if not confidently anticipated. The good results which have followed the modern treatment of peritonitis by laparotomy and irrigation tend to support this view, and it is, I believe, by carrying out the principle I have feebly indicated that such successes are to be explained. In support of this view I would allude again to the partial withdrawal of fluid from tense cavities for the relief of tension, and the result which commonly follows the practice, for it cannot but be acknowledged that this action is often speedily followed by the absorption of the liquid which is left, and recovery from the local trouble. The partial withdrawal of pent-up fluids apparently so frees the venous, lymphatic and arterial circulation of parts which have by the pressure been previously embarrassed, as to be followed by their full physiological action and the progress of repair toward a cure. In many a large hæmatoma I have despaired of its absorption and a natural cure till I had withdrawn some of its serous contents and removed tension, when a rapid recovery followed.

In not a few inflamed knee-, hip-, and other joints made tense by inflammatory effusions, and so tense as to excite a fear of loss of structure, has a rapid recovery followed a careful aspiration sufficient to relieve tension, or a subcutaneous puncture of the joint. Even in large abscesses, and particularly chronic abscesses, the same result may be chronicled, that is, the rapid absorption of what may have been left in the abscess cavity after the withdrawal of only a part. And the explanation of these results can probably be found in what has been already said.

I have thus, Mr. President, laid before you—although, I fear imperfectly—many, if not most, of the clinical data connected with what has been called tension, or centrifugal pressure. I have pointed out its causes and its effects, and more partienlarly the great value of pain as a significant sign of most forms of tension, and especially of inflammatory tension. I have attempted also to bring out from these facts a certain principle of practice, the value of which I do not think I have exaggerated. If I were to test the value of the practical principle I have brought before you by my own personal experience, I should place it very high, for I can assure you that I have for years acted upon it and not found it wanting. To carry it out fully, we must, however, return to former lines of treatment, and employ more frequently than we do the practice of leeching in local and comparatively superficial inflammations, and of puncturing, incising, drilling, and trephining in bony and subfascial inflammations; and these means should be employed early in every case. Should we employ counter-irritation, we shall do so on a kind of principle which is intelligible, and we shall therefore be more likely to employ our measures with success. To illustrate, however, what I have said to-day more fully and completely, I must go to the diseases of the bones and periosteum; and it is to these that I hope to draw your attention in my next lecture.

LECTURE II.

ON THE EFFECTS OF TENSION, AS ILLUSTRATED IN INFLAMMATION OF BONE AND ITS TREATMENT.

MY last lecture was devoted to the subject of tension generally, and I trust I was able, with sufficient clearness, to satisfy you that tension of tissues has a widely spreading influence on the progress of disease, particularly of inflammatory disease. I pointed out what seemed to me very clear, that tension is a common factor of pain, and that in all inflammatory affections the pain of tension is not only a significant symptom of its presence, but a fair measure of its intensity. I showed how tension may and frequently does originate inflammatory action, more particularly in wounds, and that this effect takes place under every form of wound dressing. I demonstrated how in the soft tissues of the body, acute tension or tension acting at a high level, and allowed to take its course, always ends in the destruction of the tissues implicated; and pointed out that where tension was acting for any time at a low level in either hard or soft tissues, permanent change of structure, tending toward their destruction, may be looked for; and I concluded that the most satisfactory and certain method of arresting acute as well as chronic inflammatory processes is by relieving tension.

In my present lecture I hope to enforce all these conclusions by considering the effects of tension in bone when in a state of inflammation, and I do so in the belief that it is in the inflammation of bone and its fibrous covering that the effects as well as the treatment are best illustrated. The key to this conclusion is probably to be found in the vascular supply to the bone, and it will therefore be well to devote a few moments to its consideration. I have no intention, however, to weary you with any long anatomical description of bone and its covering. For our present purpose it is sufficient that we recognize the close vascular connection which exists between the compact tissue of bone and its periosteal envelope, as well as the free anastomosis of the vessels which supply the medullary canal of bone with those of its compact substance. It is likewise important to keep in view that this vascular connection applies as much to its venous as to its arterial supply. The arrangement of the capillaries of the bone also must not be forgotten, for these pass through fine bony canals, which are incapable of dilatation or contraction, and flow into veins similarly arranged. The veins, moreover, have pouch-like dilatations or sinuses in their course, are deficient in muscular fibres and valves, and in all such internal arrangements and external surroundings as in the softer structures help toward the free circulation of the blood. In fact, the circulatory system in bones is so arranged as to favor blood stasis. With such anatomical arrangements it becomes, therefore, clearly intelligible why an inflammatory action which may have originated in one part of the bone—let us say in the endosteum—so soon involves the outside compact bone structures; why inflammation of the periosteum which envelops the bone is so frequently complicated with inflammation of the bone itself; and, last but not least, why when bone is inflamed and there is the necessary slowing of the blood current through the capillaries and veins of the inflamed parts, it is as rare as it must be difficult for natural powers, unaided by art, to bring about a cure. Thus it is, therefore, that we find, when acute inflammation attacks the periosteum, that death of the bone from extension of the inflammatory process is a common consequence; that acute inflammation of the medullary cavity of a bone (osteo-myelitis, endostitis, ostitis), as a rule, spreads to its compact walls, and ends in more or less destruction of the bone; and that, where this result does not follow, the formation of abscess or abscesses in the affected bone, with partial necrosis, is the termination to be expected. For when an acute inflammation has attacked a bone, whether as an extension from the periosteum or otherwise, its termination may be either in necrosis, partial or complete, or in the formation of an acute abscess or abscesses; the abscess cavity containing not only pus with the molecularly destroyed bone tissue, but as often as not a distinct sequestrum; for molar and molecular death of tissue with suppuration are the common results of acute inflammation of bone as of softer structures.

If we pass on to consider the effects of *chronic inflammation of bone*, the same want of recovery by resolution has to be recorded, with the same tendency for the inflammatory action to bring about destructive changes. An inflammatory process, once started, goes on slowly but surely, although possibly with intervals of relief and exacerbations; but it ends either in some abscess in the bone, the death of a small portion of bone with the condensation of more, or the sclerosing of the whole bone. Examples of all these terminations are both numerous and good in our own and other museums. It may be added, however, that where sclerosis of bone is met with, there is usually some degree of destruction of bone associated with it, either in the shape of limited necrosis or abscess; and I have reason to believe that if all apparently merely sclerosed bones were carefully divided into sections, either a small necrosed sequestrum or chronic abscess in the bone would be very generally discovered, the sclerosing process being due to persistent irritation kept up by the abscess or sequestrum. I have frequently myself found this, and conse·quently acted upon the knowledge, and I may add with advantage. In a case to be recorded later on, this fact is well illustrated, and in another case under Mr. Cock, which took place in 1856, in which the limb of a man, aged thirty seven, was amputated high up in the thigh for enormous enlargement of the femur of many years' standing, and in which the bone was like ivory, a very small piece of necrosed bone was found in its central canal, unattended by any external suppuration.

To find a full explanation of this fact—that inflamed bone and its periosteal covering, as a rule, ends in some destructive change—we must go to tension, for by universal consent surgeons acknowledge that the death of an acutely inflamed bone is brought about by such a cause, and also, that the intense pain which is connected with it, is without doubt, due to the inability of the bone tissue to yield in any degree to the distending influence of inflammatory hyperæmia and its consequences. And I trust I may find many to share with me the belief that it is this same tension in subacute and chronic inflammation of bone which not only keeps up the process and prevents recovery by resolution from taking place, but also tends to bring about the destructive and sclerosing changes in bone with which we are all familiar. Why it is that, in bone, tension in any of its degrees is so fruitful of harm, must be explained by the anatomical facts relating to its circulation to which I have drawn your attention, and the difficulty under which unaided natural processes must consequently labor to enable the circulation of the bone to overcome the tendency to capillary blood stasis which forms the essential pathological phenomenon of inflammation, and upon which the life or death of the bone depends. For in bone, as there are neither in the normal arrangement of its capillaries and veins, nor in its surroundings, any such provisions as are found in soft tissues to favor the flow of blood in its usual physiological condition, so under the influence of disease, and more particularly of inflammation, in which the slowing of the blood current and capillary blood stasis are the invariable consequences, the difficulty of restoring the circulation to its normal condition must of necessity be infinitely greater. Under these circumstances the practical inference to be drawn is this—that it is the surgeon's duty, without reserve, when inflammation of bone and its covering can be made out to exist, to do what lies in his art to relieve tension; and it will be my object in this lecture to enforce this view.

As a preliminary point of great importance, however, I would draw your attention to the value of pain as an indication of the presence of inflammation of bone, such pain appearing to me to be the result of tension under all circumstances. In acute disease this is admitted by universal consent, and in the more chronic forms it has a no less general influence. The pain in its nature may not always be severe, or in the bulk of cases capable of being described as more than an ache, but this ache will probably at times be intensified by walking if the trouble be in the lower extremity, or by hanging the arm down during the day if in the upper limb—by anything, in fact, that helps blood stasis in the part. It is also, always, worse at night, when the circulation of the blood through the part with that of the body generally is encouraged by the warmth of bed; indeed, at these times the pain may be severe —very severe. Such pains in bone, increased at night, have been commonly believed to be associated with syphilis, and have been called osteo-copic pains. Such a conclusion may, however, be wrong. The pains, nevertheless, are always bone pains, and as a rule due to inflammation. Occasionally, indeed generally, there is increased local heat in the bone affected, although in deeply placed bones there may be a difficulty in detecting it. In such a bone as the tibia the increased heat which is present is very marked if rightly tested; and what I man by the term "rightly" is as follows. The limb should be exposed with its fellow for purposes of comparison, and the palm of the surgeon's hand placed—if the suspected inflamed bone be the tibia—above the knee-joint, and allowed to rest there for a few seconds to appreciate the normal temperature. The hand should then be passed *slowly* downward over the suspected bone, say, to the ankle; and during this action any increase in local temperature, even if localized to the space of . half-a-crown or less, may be at once detected. The sound limb should then be examined in the same way, and the sensations acquired by the two hands compared. The test takes less time to make than it has taken me to describe. It is far better than simply grasping the suspected bone with one hand and the sound one with the other, the method in which the examination is usually conducted. By the same method, even if the femur be the bone affected, the increase in temperature can be detected. I trust I may be pardoned for this digression. I have, however, no desire to enter into the diagnosis of these cases generally, and have dwelt upon the diagnostic value of pain more to draw your attention to its use as indicating the presence of inflammatory tension in bone than for any other purpose, for my object is to show you that this tension must be relieved, if any help toward cure can be entertained. To a certain extent most surgeons recognize the truth of these remarks, and more particularly in their treatment of acute periosteal inflammation. For they not only act upon the principle I am anxious to enforce, but also teach their pupils to make an incision down to bone as soon as the diagnosis of acute periostitis is sufficiently definite. This incision is called for primarily with a view of relieving subperiosteal tension and the hyperæmia of the probably involved bone; and secondarily, in oder to guard against the dangers, which should always be recognized, of the inflammatory effusions burrowing beneath the periosteal coverings of the epiphyses, or through the epiphyses themselves into the neighboring joints, and so originating a suppurative synovitis. No words that I can use would be too strong to support this practice, for it is without doubt the only reasonable one.

When acute ostitis, endostitis, or osteo-myelitis attacks the shaft of a long bone, and still more when it originates in the juxta-epiphyseal cartilage or in the epiphysis itself, the necessity of making a free external incision is likewise a fairly well recognized practice. It is here adopted for the same reasons as have rendered it necessary in acute periosteal inflammations; but in these cases it should be regarded as a means only to a more important end—that is, to give room for the surgeon to relieve the tension in the bone itself, either by drilling, trephining, or otherwise freely exposing the centre of the bone in which the inflammation originated, or to which it may have spread. This operation is doubtless the only one which acts favorably upon the disease, in either arresting its course or limiting its destructive tendencies. But I would wish to go a step farther and urge that active local means to relieve tension should, as a principle of practice, always be immediately taken when such has been brought about by acute inflammatory processes, whether the periosteum or endosteum be its primary seat; and that the surgeon need not, before he acts upon this principle, wait, and in so doing lose valuable time, while a definite or exact diagnosis is being made. In-deed, in a clinical point of view, acute periostitis and endostitis had better be regarded as identical affections, since in both there is, pathologically, rapid effusion and extreme tension of tissue, which very quickly bring about its death, and, clinically, deep swelling, severe local pain, and marked constitutional disturbance. The general symptoms are frequently so severe as to raise the suspicion of the patient being the subject of an acute general rheumatic rather than of an acute local affection, as proved by the fact that in hospital practice many of these cases are primarily admitted into the physicians' rather than the surgeons' wards. Should joint symptoms coexist with acute epiphyseal inflammation, or follow diaphyseal ostitis as a result of burrowing of the inflammatory fluids beneath the periosteum into the joint, the surgeon should act more energetically, and he need not despair of seeing the joint symptoms disappear if relief can be afforded to the inflammation in the bone and a vent given to inflammatory products. If the joint has not suppurated, a perfect recovery may be anticipated; but if this consequence has ensued, a recovery with ankylosis should be expected. The surgeon should remember that the destructive effects of tension in acute periostitis or endostitis is in most cases worked out within a week from the onset of the inflammation, so that, if good is to be gained by treatment, it is all-important that such should be applied early. He should likewise recognize the fact that by drilling or trephining inflamed bone necrosis is not produced; the operation may fail in preventing such a result taking place, but it will invariably tend toward its prevention and limitation. The incision down to bone in acute inflammation of the periosteum cannot be made too early; and in acute ostitis the same incision made as a preliminary measure to enable the surgeon to drill, trephine, or lay open the bone cavity itself, should evidence of its inflammation be present, can only tend toward good. If the periosteal incision be made in the early stage, in which blood-stained serum or blood alone is effused beneath the periosteum, the surgeon may entertain a reasonable hope that recovery will take place without necrosis; but if pus be present the chances are that more or less death of bone will ensue. In exceptional cases, however, a better result may be obtained. The following case of hemorrhagic acute periostitis very forcibly illustrates all · these points, with others, and is consequently worthy of atten-tion.

CASE X.—A boy aged nine came under my care in Novem-ber, 1876, with symptoms of acute inflammation of the bones of the left leg and ankle, as indicated by great swelling, red-ness, and tension of the soft tissues over the bones, and intense pain in the part. His temperature was 104°, pulse 140. These symptoms were said to have followed a kick received three days previously. As soon as I saw him a free incision was made over the fibula, where the tension seemed to be the greatest, and the periosteum was opened with a distinct ex-plosive sound, the fluid from beneath being scattered in all directions. This fluid was, however, pure blood, clots being subsequently syringed or washed away. The bone was com-pletely stripped of its periosteal covering. Two months later a large piece of necrosed bone exfoliated and was removed from the fibula, and the limb recovered. On the fourth day after the boy's admission into the hospital with acute perios-titis of the left fibula, which had been attributed to a kick, the right leg became affected in precisely the same way; the temperature rose to 102.6°; the pulse to 144. The affection was treated by a free incision over the fibula, as in the other limb, but within twenty-four hours of the onset of the symptoms, and blood escaped with the same explosive sound as on the former occasion from beneath the periosteum, and the bone was left freely exposed. No necrosis, however, ensued. Five days after his admission it was evident that the periosteum of the tibia of the right leg was involved with the fibula, and an incision was made directly down to the bone, from which pus freely escaped. The local and constitutional symptoms at once subsided, but necrosis of the tibia subsequently followed, and a sequestrum was removed at the end of two months. A good recovery afterward took place. In this case it is worthy of note that in the acute inflammation of the periosteum of the fibula, which came on while the boy was in bed, and was treated within twenty-four hours of the onset of symptoms by a deep incision, no necrosis followed. In the opposite limb, where the same trouble attacked the same bone and the incision was not made till the third day, necrosis ensued; and in the tibia, where suppuration was allowed to take place before the tension was relieved, the same result had to be recorded. The fluid that was effused beneath the periosteum of both fibulæ was blood, and in both limbs the tension of the periosteum was so great that its incision was attended with an explosive sound. No better case could be brought before you to illustrate the value of an early and free relief of local tension than the one I have briefly read, and certainly no better example could illustrate the benefit of action and early treatment in checking and limiting disease.

In the following two cases the periosteal incision was not made until suppuration had occurred; but in neither of them did necrosis follow. Such a possibility is consequently a strong inducement for the surgeon to interfere, even in cases which are unpromising.

Case XI.—A boy aged ten (David K——) came under my care in July, 1877, with his left thigh and knee-joint enormously swollen, tense, and tender. He was also in a state of high fever, with a temperature of 101.2°. The local trouble had come on two days previously, with pain and swelling, and this had followed a fall upon the knee two days earlier. The diagnosis made was acute femoral periostitis, with effusion into the knee-joint from contiguity. An incision was therefore made into the outer side of the thigh, between the tendon of the biceps and ilio-tibial fascial band, down to the femur, when six or more ounces of pus escaped, the femur being found stripped of its periosteal covering for some inches. The abscess cavity was washed out and drained. Great and immediate relief followed this operation, and a steady convalescence in about six weeks. There was no dead bone as a result of the inflammation, although pus had formed in two days from the origin of the trouble.

CASE XII.—In this case a like favorable result took place. A boy aged four (W. P——) came under my care in 1876, with a deep-seated, tender, and painful swelling involving the centre of the left femur, which had speedily followed a fall downstairs nineteen days previously. Pain and swelling had appeared a day or so after the fall; but for a week the child limped about, although he was ill. When I saw him a deep periosteal abscess evidently existed, which I laid open, evacuating pus and exposing bone. Rapid recovery ensued, and without loss of tissue.

If I am not wearying you, I should like to quote the leading facts of other cases, in which acute inflammation attacked the epiphyses of bone, or the diaphyseal cartilage; in which by a like treatment good results were secured.

CASE XIII. *Acute Necrosis of the Head of the Tibia, with Inflammation of the Joint; Opening of the Abscess in the Bone, and Removal of a Sequestrum; Rapid Recovery.*— Robert G——, aged nine, came under my care at Guy's Hospital on October 4th, 1887, with acute periostitis or ostitis of the head of the left tibia, which had followed closely upon a blow he had received when running seven days previously in a fall upon the knee against a curbstone. The accident was followed by pain, which became severe on the second day, when swelling appeared. He could not then walk. When admitted on the fifth day of the symptoms, there was effusion into the knee-joint, extreme pain on movement, and tenderness, but no fluctuation over the head of the tibia. His temperature was 102.6°. An incision was at once made down to the bone, but blood alone escaped. This operation, however, gave relief, but only for a time. Consequently a second incision was made on the inner side of the bone, and later on others, for diffused suppuration took place all round the head of the bone, which suggested more than the possibility that an abscess existed in the bone with more or less necrosis. On January 1st the bone was consequently explored by means of an incision and chisel, and a large cavity in the head of the tibia exposed, in which rested a sequestrum. This was then removed, and the cavity well cleansed with sponges dipped in hot iodine water. The bone left seemed to be a mere shell, the *upper surface of which formed the articular facet of the joint.* The cavity in the bone was then allowed to fill with blood, and iodoform dressing was applied over the wound, with a sponge as a pad and the whole limb was fixed on a posterior splint. All constitutional symptoms rapidly disappeared after this operation. The wound quickly filled up, and in six weeks the boy was practically well. In another three weeks he was allowed to move the knee, when the movements became natural. By the end of March he was quite well, and left the hospital with a perfectly movable knee-joint. In this case an earlier expioration of the bone should doubtless have been made. Such a measure would probably have limited the disease, and would certainly have saved pain.

CASE XIV. *Acute Abscess, with Necrosis in the Head of the Tibia; free Incision into the Bone; Removal of Sequestrum; Recovery.*—George H——, aged fifteen, a healthy boy, came under my care in July, 1875, with a tensely swollen and inflamed left leg below the knee, and a discharging sinus over the inner tuberosity of the tibia. The boy was in great pain, and was very ill with high fever. The swelling had been present for three weeks, and had followed a blow below the knee. An abscess over the head of the tibia had been opened two days previously. As there was not sufficient drainage for the abscess, a free incision was at once made over the head of the tibia, and the parts were irrigated. A fistulous opening was then discovered leading into the bone; this was at once enlarged, when a cavity in the head of the bone the size of a walnut and lined with membrane, was exposed. The cavity contained a rounded sequestrum, which was removed, while the cavity of the abscess was cleansed. After this procedure rapid recovery ensued, and the boy left the hospital on August 30th, well, with a sound limb and movable knee-joint.

The following cases, kindly furnished to me by my colleague, Mr. Davies-Colley, further illustrate this point.

CASE XV. *Drilling for Acute Necrosis of Tibia; Suppuration of Knee-joint; Incision into Joint; Recovery, with Movable Knee.*—Percy C. C——, aged nearly four, was admitted into Guy's Hospital on March 16th, 1885, with acute inflammation of the right tibia. On the 11th his leg had begun to be painful. His father said that no cause was known, but on a subsequent occasion he told us the boy had had a fall the same day or a day or two before, and that he had some fits before the knee pain began. On admission the boy's temperature was 102.8°. Fluctuation was felt over the whole of the subcutaneous portion of the right tibia. Free incisions were made down to the bone, which was found to be nearly all bare, and was drilled in four places, whence pus welled out. On April 27th the patient's temperature was 105°. On the 30th of that month the right knee-joint was swollen and fluctuating. Free incisions into the joint were made, giving exit to thick curdy pus. At the same time the whole of the anterior part of the diaphysis of the tibia was removed. The boy recovered, with a perfectly movable knee-joint.

CASE XVI. *Acute Necrosis of the Lower Half of the Tibia; Suppuration of the Ankle-joint; Drilling of Bone and Incision into Joint: Recovery.*—Fred. D——, aged sixteen, was admitted on May 12th, 1882. He had been a little out of sorts; had fallen and hurt his left ankle. Œdema of the leg and high temperature followed. On May 18th a free incision was made down to the tibia in its lower third; the ankle-joint, which was suppurating, was also opened. On May 23d the temperature, which had at first fallen, had again risen; and the patient had had some vomiting. Some swelling was found just below the tubercle of the tibia. Ether was again administered, and pus evacuated by a free incision. The bone was then drilled, when two or three drops of pus oozed out from the drill holes. From the fact that the second periosteal abcess was separated from the first by apparently healthy bone, Mr. Davies-Colley thought that the disease had extended from one part of the bone to the other by suppuration along the medullary cavity, and that it was desirable to give exit to the pent-up pus. After necrosis of nearly the whole shaft, the boy went out quite well, with a stiff ankle. Mr. Davies-Colley remarks: "If I had drilled when I cut down upon the lower third of the limb, I might have prevented the extensive necrosis. So I determined in future cases to drill earlier."

CASE XVII. *Subacute Inflammation of the Tibia; Incision down to the Bone; Abscess in the Bone; Subsequent Recovery.*—Martha F——, aged fourteen, was admitted on July 16th, 1882. She had injured her left ankle a week previously. There was swelling of the ankle and over the lower half of the leg, and semi-fluctuation over the tibia. A free incision was made, but only serum came away; the periosteum was not separated. On September 22d a sinus was still left. An incision was then made down to the bone, which was found to be enlarged, and converted into a cavity containing pus, lymph, and small sequestra, which had to be scraped away. The patient was discharged convalescent on November 21st, 1882.

Of the foregoing case Mr. Davies-Colley remarks: "If I had drilled at the first operation I should very likely have saved her a long illness and some danger."

If this practice were carried out systematically in all cases of acute inflammation of bone and its covering, I do not believe we should hear so much as we do of subperiosteal resection of the shafts of inflamed bones—an operation I have never done, nor seen to be needed; and amputation for acute endostitis would only be called for in neglected cases, or where joint complication rendered any partial measure impossible. At any rate, it may be safely said that the necessity for either of these severe measures would rarely occur. In any local periosteal inflammation, in which symptoms are less severe than in the cases quoted, the same principle of practice is equally applicable, and, it may be added, beneficial. Thus in my own practice I have, with invariable advantage, in not a few examples of local periostitis, where local pain was a serious symptom, made a free subcutaneous incision down to the bone through the inflamed periosteum by means of a tenotomy knife carefully introduced through a valvular opening in the skin; the incision not only relieved tension, the cause of pain, but at the same time checked inflammatory action. Where this little operation is done early, before suppuration has taken place or the vitality of the bone has been jeopardized, a rapid recovery may be looked for; and where more serious structural changes have taken place, pain is relieved, and, there is reason to believe, the destructive changes are limited. In the local periostitis or ostitis of a cranial bone, with or without fracture, this detail of practice cannot be too speedily carried out; but in these cases an open incision is probably to be preferred. In the following case the benefit of the treatment was well exemplified.

CASE XVIII.—*Periostitis of both Tibiæ after Typhoid Fever; Suppuration of one Limb and Necrosis; Subcutaneous Division of the Periosteum of the other; Recovery.*—In March, 1865, I was consulted by Mr. B——, aged twenty-six, for some great thickening of the shafts of both tibiæ, which had appeared seven weeks previously when he was recovering from typhoid fever. There was much pain in both limbs, and in the right apparently suppuration, but not in the left, which was hard to the touch and very painful. The swelling over the right tibia was laid open by a free incision, and pus evacuated, the bone beneath being evidently necrosed. The swelling on the left limb was divided subcutaneously down to the bone by means of a long tenotomy knife; blood alone escaped. Pain was at once relieved, and did not return; and a rapid recovery took place. In the right limb some dead bone was eventually removed, and recovery followed.

Having thus far considered the effects of tension acting at a high level in acute inflammation of the periosteum and bone, and dwelt upon the principle of practice which should be acted

upon for its relief, with the best means of carrying it out, I
propose now to pass on and consider the effects of tension in
the more chronic and subacute affections of the same structures; and trust that I may be able to convince you that it is
by acting upon the same practical principle that the best hope
can be entertained of arresting the inflammatory action and
of placing the inflamed part in the most favorable condition
for repair.   To allow these cases to take their course, every
surgeon will admit, is most unsatisfactory; for their course
is a long one, often for years; and they commonly, if not invariably, end in either local suppuration, local necrosis, or
sclerosis of bone, but rarely in recovery by resolution; and in
any individual case one or more of these results may be found
together.   The preparations before me demonstrate the truth
of these remarks.   The object of the surgeon in the treatment
of these cases should therefore be to anticipate these organic
changes, and prevent them where he can.   Attempts to do
this by medicinal and local measures, other than operative,
are neither hopeful nor successful, although the value of the
iodides and of mercury in certain cases must be recognized;
and I feel confident that the only sound principle of practice
which should be carried out in examples of chronic ostitis is
the one based on the relief of tension, as indicated by pain.
To illustrate my meaning better, let me place before you a
typical and not uncommon case.   A surgeon has before him a
patient, usually a child or young adult, who complains of a
dull, aching, stubborn pain, localized in the shaft, or more
commonly in the extremity of a long bone.   The pain has
probably existed off and on for months, or possibly for years,
and it is to a degree constant; it tends, as John Hunter expressed it, "rather to produce sickness than to rouse."   After
exercise, or use of the affected limb, the pain is intensified,
sometimes to a high degree, and at night, when the patient
is warm in bed, it is to a certainty aggravated.   In the subacute cases fever or febrile disturbance may exist; in the more
chronic cases it is rarely met with.   On local examination,
there is probably, if the affection has been of some standing,
an enlargement of the bone, and on passing the palm of the
hand from above downward over the seat of mischief an increase of temperature is to be detected.   Firm local pressure
recognizes in some cases a tender spot, while in others local

percussion through the surgeon's finger elicits pain. There may or may not have been a history of some local injury months or years previously. There may or may not be some general symptoms; as a rule, the general symptoms are conspicuous by their absence. In such a case as this the only diagnosis that can be made is one of inflammation of the bone, which has been persistent and progressive; but whether the case be one of osteo-myelitis of the articular extremity of the bone, as one author might like to call it, or of rarefying osteitis, as modern authorities would describe it, is of small importance. In simple pathological language, the case is one of inflammation of the shaft of the bone, or of the cancellous bone situated at the epiphyseal extremity of the diaphysis (juxta-epiphyseal ostitis), or of the epiphysis itself, which experience tells us in no uncertain tone, if it be allowed to continue, will end in some destructive change, with more or less condensation of bone structure. What change the bone may have undergone at the time when it came under observation must be a dark point, and one quite beyond the power of the surgeon to diagnose with any certainty. There is happily, however, no great necessity for the surgeon before he acts to form any very definite diagnosis upon these points. He need do no more than recognize the presence of inflammation in the bone, and of tension as indicated by pain, to induce him to take steps for its relief; and a very little experience will prove to him that by the relief of tension in the bone, wherever it may be found, pain will be relieved, if not made to disappear, and with its amelioration the inflammatory process will probably subside. Under the circumstances now being considered, I should at once make an incision down to the bone through the periosteum, and perforate the bone with a drill, well into its centre in one or more points, according to the extent of bone involved; and I should do this with the object of relieving tension in the bone. If blood alone or serum escaped from the punctured wound, I should conclude that no destructive changes had taken place in the bone, and consequently I should do no more, in the confidence that the simple operation I had performed would, in all probability, be followed by the immediate and permanent loss of pain—which, it is to be remembered, is the measure of tension—and by the cure of the disease by resolution. Should, however, the local pain persist after this operation, I should drill again; and if this measure proved unsuccessful, I should infer that in all probability some abscess cavity is present which must be sought for. The trephine under these circumstances would be the right instrument to employ with the drill as a bone-searcher introduced through the trephine excavation. Should pus or puriform fluid escape from the drill opening made in my first exploration, I should have recourse at once to the use of the trephine, cutting forceps, saw, or chisel, with the view, not only of making room for a full exploration of the abscess cavity, but also for the removal of any sequestrum which might be present in the cavity; and last, but not least, the cavity itself should be thoroughly wiped out and cleared of all lymph, caseating pus or old inflammatory material, which if left would do harm. In subacute and chronic ostitis, the single inducement which should lead the surgeon to interfere is deep-seated pain, and particularly nocturnal pain; for the pain not only clearly indicates tension of the inflamed tissues, but also suggests steady progress of the trouble. All experience shows that in these cases, inflammation continues until relief to tension be found either by the destructive processes of the disease itself or by the surgeon's art. The following brief notes of cases well illustrate the practice I have sketched out, with its results.

CASE XIX. *Ostitis of the Head of the Tibia Cured by Drilling.*—George S——, aged thirty, came into my hands for treatment on April 5th, 1871, with great enlargement of the head of the left tibia. The trouble had appeared about four months previously, with pain, and it had followed a blow. The pain was constant, and of a dull aching kind; it was far worse at night. The knee-joint was unaffected, and the soft parts over the bone appeared to be natural. There was no history of syphilis. The diagnosis of ostitis having been arrived at, I made an incision down to the bone, and in so doing found the periosteum much thickened. I then drilled the head of the tibia in two places, and from the openings in the bone blood alone escaped. The operation was followed by immediate relief, and pain did not return. The bone gradually diminished in size. The wound healed kindly in a month, and the man left the hospital well in six weeks. Some months later he was at work with a sound limb.

CASE XX. *Abscess in the Shaft of the Fibula, Drilled and then Trephined; Cure.*—Frank R——, aged twenty-eight, a healthy commercial traveller, who had never had syphilis, came into Guy's under my care in January, 1885, with a hard, painful swelling over the centre of his right fibula, and some œdema of the foot and parts around. There was locally increased heat. The swelling had been gradually coming on for four months, and it appeared with pain. The pain had been constant since, although it was worse at times, and invariably so at night. On several occasions he had had to lie by, and for three months had gone about on crutches. An incision was made down to the fibula through the peronei muscles, which were found to be infiltrated with inflammatory material. The periosteum over the bone was thickened. I drilled the bone in two places, and from each opening pus exuded. I consequently trephined the bone, and exposed a cavity from which at least an ounce of pus escaped. There was no sequestrum in the cavity. The cavity was washed out with iodine water, cleaned thoroughly with sponge, and dressed with iodoform gauze, etc., and within six weeks the man was well.

CASE XXI. *Abscess in the Head of the Tibia Following a Blow, which Discharged into the Popliteal Space; Free Opening into the Bone; Recovery.*—Robert J——, aged forty-three, came under my care in July, 1869, with his left leg flexed upon his thigh, a discharging sinus in the popliteal space, and marked expansion of the head of the left tibia. There was constant pain in the bone, and three inches below the knee firm pressure could not be borne. Twenty-five years previously he had had ostitis of the tibia, followed by the exfoliation of bone six months later and recovery. He remained well for twenty years, when he received a blow upon the inner side of his knee, which was followed by a popliteal abscess. For the previous nine months his leg had been gradually becoming flexed upon the thigh. The case was regarded as one of abscess in the upper part of the tibia discharging into the popliteal space. Under these circumstances, the abscess in the bone was opened by means of a strong knife, the bone being thin, and about an inch of the abscess wall in the bone was removed. A large cavity was thus exposed, which extended upward toward the knee-joint. The cavity was lined with granulations, and contained pus, but no dead bone. It had evidently opened into the popliteal space. The cavity was well washed out, with the popliteal abscess. The knee was extended, and the whole limb fixed upon a posterior splint. The wound was dressed carefully with dry dressing. Subsequently repair went on uninterruptedly. The cavity in the bone filled up; all pain ceased; the popliteal abscess rapidly closed; and by August 12th—that is, five weeks after the operation—the man was convalescent and the wound had healed. A month later the cure was complete.

CASE XXII. *Chronic Ostitis of the Distal Ends of the Tibia and Fibula, after a Compound Fracture of the Bones;*

*Great Expansion of Bones; Drilling of Bones, with Rapid
Recovery.*—Herbert G——, aged twenty-four, came under my
care on June 9th, 1886, with a compound comminuted fracture
of the tibia and fibula, about four inches above the ankle joint.
He did well after the accident, and left the hospital on August
6th, with a protective splint, convalescent. Four months later
he returned, with great enlargement of the distal ends of the
broken bones and much local pain, which was aggravated by
exercise or pressure. There was likewise increase of heat in
the part. The foot was raised and fixed upon a splint, and
cold applied by means of Leiter's coil, with some benefit and
relief to pain. He then left the hospital, but returned on February 7th worse than ever—that is, the bones were expanded
and more painful, and the pain was worse at night. The general appearance of the ankle suggested the presence of some
new growth. On March 4th, 1887, I made a free incision down
to the tibia over the enlarged and inflamed bone, and then
drilled the bone, when blood alone escaped from the wound.
The operation was followed by immediate relief and the steady
diminution of the swollen bone. On March 28th the same
operation was performed upon the lower end of the fibula,
with a like result. The man left the hospital, well, on May
5th, and reported himself three months later as quite well.

CASE XXIII. *Ostitis and Central Abscess, following
Fracture of the Shaft of the Humerus Twenty Years Before;
Drilling and Trephining; Recovery.*—George W——, aged
twenty-seven, was admitted into Guy's Hospital under Mr.
Davies-Colley, in November, 1885, with pain in the lower part
of the arm, thickening of the lower end of the shaft of the
humerus, and a small sinus three inches above the olecranon.
He had received a simple fracture of the humerus twenty years
previously. For six years he had remained well; then, from
time to time, there had been a discharge of spicula of dead
bone. There was good movement of the elbow joint. On November 17th, the patient being etherized, Mr. Davies-Colley
made an incision down on the back of the lower three inches of
the humerus, which were thickened and rough. A small cloaca
existed at the upper part of the olecranon fossa. The back of
the humerus was drilled three inches up, where the sinus was,
and where he had complained of much tenderness. A cylin-
drical abscess cavity was exposed and Mr. Davies-Colley removed by a trephine, etc., nearly all its posterior wall. It was
three inches long by three quarters of an inch in diameter, and
communicated with the small cloaca in the olecranon fossa.
There was no sequestrum in it. He recovered rapidly.

This clearing of the abscess cavity after its evacuation, or
the removal of a sequestrum, is best done by sponge. A piece
of sponge on dressing forceps acts as a fine raspatory on a

bone cavity, and cleanses it more thoroughly of all inflammatory products and molecular fragments of necrosed bone, than
anything else. It is far better than scraping or gouging the
bone. The sponge I have dipped ın hot iodine water before
use. When the cavity has been well cleared out, and no foreign .body in the shape of necrosed bone is left behind, a recovery with a good limb may be expected to result. After the
operation described I leave the case much to nature, but take
great care to keep the wound aseptic and the parts involved
perfectly immovable. If the cavity fills up with blood-clot I
do not disturb it, but keep its surface dusted with boracic acid
and iodoform powder, and covered with a simple dressing of
iodoform gauze dipped in terebene and oil. In the daily dressing, iodine water is employed to irrigate the wound. By these
means I have had many cases in which the cavity rapidly filled
up with granulation tissue, beneath and within the blood-clot,
and subsequently cicatrized without any trouble; the presence
of the blood-clot, kept aseptic, doubtless much helping—in
ways I need not stop to consider—the growth and organiza-
tion of granulation tissue. Some of these cases have been in
subjects who were feeble, and who might have been called
tuberculous, and yet in them repair went on as favorably as
in the apparently more robust. Where with inflammation of
the articular extremity of a bone—whether originating in an
epiphysis, diaphysis, or intervening cartilage—the joint itself
is implicated, the case has of necessity a far more serious as-
peet. And the fact should at once lead the surgeon to be more
energetic in his treatment, rather than dilatory; for if the
joint complication shows itself only as a subacute or chronic
synovitis, such a complication may be expected to subside, if
its cause, the bone inflammation, be relieved. In the following case the truth of these observations is well illustrated.

CASE XXIV. *Chronic Ostitis of the Head of the Tibia,
with Joint Symptoms; Drilling of Bone; Recovery.*—Henry
R——, a master butcher, aged twenty-eight, came under my
care in October, 1887, with some enlargement of the head of the
right tibia, and a constant aching pain in the part. The pain
had existed for *ten* years, having originated when he was eighteen, and had come on without any known cause. Every few
months he had been quite incapacitated. At times the soft parts
over the bone swelled, particularly after violent exercise. The
pain likewise then became much aggravated, preventing sleep;

also, it was always worse at night. The knee joint had been stiff for some months, any attempt to flex it exciting pain. There as no history of syphilis. On admission, there was impaired movement in the knee joint, and some swelling. There was very evident enlargement of the head of the tibia, and more particularly about its inner tuberosity. The leg at this part measured nearly an inch more in circumference than its fellow. At one spot there was increased tenderness over the bone, and the soft parts covering it were slightly thickened. The diagnosis was chronic inflammation of the bone. I accordingly made an incision over the painful spot, and reflected a thickened periosteum. I then drilled the bone well into its centre. Blood alone escaped. I made only one puncture into the bone, as I was anxious to test its efficacy, but was prepared to do more should relief not be afforded. The wound, which I left as an open one, was dressed with care, and the limb fixed on a splint. Everything went on well. All pain ceased after the operation, never to return; and the wound healed in a month. At the end of that time the patient was allowed to move his knee, which he did without pain; and in another month he was quite well. At the present time (five months after the operation) he is well and at work, somewhat surprised at the rapid relief he obtained for a trouble he had had so long.

CASE XXV. *Drilling for Chronic Ostitis; Recovery.*— G. A. T——, aged seventeen, was admitted to the hospital under the care of Mr. Davies-Colley, on Jan. 30th, 1884. He was a tall, thin youth, who had suffered pain in the lower end of the left tibia for two years. No cause for its origin was assigned. He was at first treated with iodide of potassium and perchloride of mercury, and with the local application of ung. hydrarg. co., but no improvement resulted. On April 30th, 1884, the tibia was drilled in eleven places to the depth of from half an inch to an inch. The bone was soft. Nothing but blood came away. On May 5th there was freedom from pain. On May 8th, as there was some pain at night, he was ordered a mixture of potassium iodide and the perchloride of mercury. On May 25th the patient was discharged cured. He had no pain and walked quite well.

CASE XXVI. *Chronic Inflammation of the Upper Third of the Tibia following a Blow Three Months Previously; Drilling; Recovery.*—Henry T—, aged thirty, a carman, married, having three children, was admitted, under Mr. Davies-Colley, on March 22d, 1876, with the upper part of the right tibia swollen. There was no redness over it, but some tenderness. There was severe pain in the bone, which was worse when he set his foot to the ground. He suffered also at night from a pain of a "jerking" character, which woke him up. The swelling had come gradually after a kick from a horse received three months before his admission. He had never had any venereal disease. He was kept in bed; ung. hydrarg. co. was applied, and iodide of potassium administered at first in three-grain and afterward in ten grain doses, three times a day. After three weeks he went out relieved; but he soon returned with the pain as bad as ever. He was again admitted on May 1st, 1876. On the 13th, an incision was made under an anæsthetic down to the tibia; and the bone was drilled with a gimlet. A week later, the wound was nearly healed and the pain had gone. The man left the hospital quite well on June 7th.

When an abscess has made its way into an articulation, the destruction of that joint is a general result, and under these circumstances amputation is often called for. To prevent this complication must ever, therefore, be a surgeon's great aim, and this can only be done either by checking the inflammatory action in the bone before suppuration and destructive changes have taken place, or by finding a vent for the external discharge of the abscess. The experience of every surgeon will supply abundant evidence of the truth of these remarks; and it would be well if we could say from the same experience that an equal number of cases could be quoted showing the advantages of early interference. Some few cases doubtless could be adduced; but I am disposed to think that too many are allowed to drift, and hopeless joint disease ensues, which has probably to be met by some trenchant operation.

CASE XXVII. *Abscess and Necrosis of the Head of the Tibia after Typhoid Fever; Removal of Bone, including a Portion of the Articular Lamella of Bone forming the Knee-joint; Recovery, with a Good Joint.*—Ada M——, aged sixteen, came under my care in June, 1884, having within three months after recovery from typhoid fever—that is, seven months before admission into Guy's—had pain in the head of the left tibia, associated with swelling and high fever, which culminated in an abscess. This has been opened, and had discharged ever since. When seen there was much effusion into the knee-joint, and a sinus existed over the inner tuberosity of the tibia, which led into a cavity in the bone, and the leg measured at the level of the sinus an inch and a half more than its fellow. The bone was consequently at once trephined and a sequestrum removed, and, while the exposed cavity was being grasped, another abscess was opened nearer the joint. The sequestrum removed included a portion of the articular surface of the tibia. The head of the bone formed a mere shell. The cavity was well syringed out with warm iodine water and dressed with iodoform gauze dipped in terebene, and the leg and knee were fixed upon a splint. When the dressings were removed on the second day, the cavity in the bone was found to be filled with blood-clot. Care was taken not to disturb this, but to keep it aseptic by washing its surface daily with iodine water, dusting it with boracic acid and iodoform powder, and dressing it as before. In six weeks the whole cavity had filled up with granulation tissue, the granulations having quietly taken the place of the blood-clot, which gradually disappeared. In another month the external wound had cicatrized, and there was movement in the joint. Six months later the limb was well and sound, with all its movements. The temperature of the patient during treatment never exceeded 99°.

CASE XXVIII. *Acute Necrosis of the Shaft of the Tibia; with Suppuration of the Knee-joint; Perforation of the Epiphysis into the Articulation; Recovery with a Stiff Joint.—* Geo. H——, aged seven years, came under my care in May, 1879, with redness and great swelling of the upper part of the right leg and œdema of the foot. The child was in intense pain, and cried on the least movement. He had a temperature of 103°, and his pulse was 125. The pain and swelling had existed for three days, and had followed a knock upon his knee against the edge of a wall two days previously. The centre of the swelling and the pain seemed to be over the inner tuberosity of the tibia. The knee-joint was enlarged. I at once made an incision down to the bone at this spot and evacuated pus from beneath the periosteum, and this measure gave relief. The knee joint, however, suppurated, and had to be incised, irrigated, and drained on June 24th; that is, about six weeks later. During these weeks the acute symptoms subsided. but it was clear that extensive necrosis of the diaphysis of the tibia had taken place; and on August 7th I removed nearly the whole of the dead shaft of the bone. Having done so, I readily found an opening which had passed through the upper epiphysis of the tibia into the knee joint, thus explaining its suppuration. In about six months the child was well, with a stiff knee.

In hip disease, secondary to bone trouble, its most common cause, the value of the practice of tapping bone is well seen, and in the following two cases well demonstrated. In one, the bone trouble had not passed beyond the hyperæmic stage; in the second, an abscess had formed and was opened. In both, good results ensued.

CASE XXIX. *Ostitis of the Trochanter and Inflammation of the Hip cured by Trephining the Bone.*—Walter S——, aged seventeen, who had enjoyed excellent health, came under my care in July, 1875, with symptoms of hip disease. They had appeared seven weeks previously as pain in the left hip when he walked, but with absence of pain when he rested, except in bed, when the pain kept him awake. The pain steadily increased and became more constant, so that at last he could not stand. On admission, the thigh on the level of the great trochanter measured an inch and a half more than its fellow. The great trochanter was much enlarged, as if from its expansion, and pressure upon it excited pain. The soft parts over the bones looked natural, but to the hand felt hotter than those over the corresponding bone. Pain was produced by movement of the bone, and on pressure into the joint behind the trochanter. I looked upon the case as one of chronic inflammation of the great trochanter and neck of the femur, with inflammation of the hip-joint from its contiguity, and I advocated tapping the bone. This I did on August 20th. I first made an incision three inches long over the trochanter down to the bone and peeled off some thickened periosteum. I then trephined the bone, which I found soft and very vasenlar. Through the trephined orifice I then drilled the bone in four directions; no pus, only blood, escaped. The wound was dressed in my usual way, and the limb fixed in a double splint. No bad symptoms followed this operation. The patient lost his pain from the date specified, his joint symptoms subsided, and the wound healed in three weeks. He left the hospital convalescent, and when seen by me some six months later he was quite well, though his hip was stiff.

CASE XXX. *Hip Disease, with Expansion of the Great Trochanter from Ostitis; Drilling of Bone, without Benefit; Trephining; Opening an Abscess in the Bone; Cure.*—A man aged forty-five came under my care in October, 1876, for hip disease of seven years' standing. He had, however, been able to get about, although with pain. Six months before coming under my care he became much worse, and was obliged to remain in bed. For some months the hip had enlarged. When admitted to the hospital his right hip was swollen, and the limb was shortened and adducted. The great trochanter was much enlarged. Movement of the limb caused pain, but the head of the femur moved smoothly in the acetabulum. Pressure over the trochanter could not be tolerated. The pain in the hip was worse at night. On October 24th the great trochanter, which was so much enlarged, was cut down upon and drilled in six places. Blood alone escaped. The bone felt soft, and was clearly vascular. No relief, but no harm, followed this operation. Consequently, on the 27th I trephined the bone, and dropped into a cavity containing lymph and pus. This was well cleared out, and its walls gouged. From this time all pain and bad symptoms disappeared, and the wound granulated. On February 28th the limb was abducted from its position of adduction, and fixed on a double splint; and by April the man was well. Three months later he could walk upon the limb without pain, although the movements of the joint were not complete.

The practice inculcated by the last two cases might, I think, be repeated more frequently with advantage.

Chronic circumscribed abscesses in bone are to be diagnosed or suspected by the presence of the same symptoms as have been given under the heading of chronic inflammation of bone generally. They are, however, often met with after many years of symptoms. In Brodie's two celebrated cases there had clearly been local evidence of bone disease for ten or twelve years respectively, about half the patient's life. These abscesses are, moreover, found in the epiphyseal extremity of a diaphysis, or in an epiphysis (a rare position). The pain of a chronic abscess in bone is, in exceptional cases, very slight; more often it is severe; it is, as other bone pain, paroxysmal and worse at night. One patient described it to me, when it was at its worst, as being "like the falling of drops of molten lead.' Others describe it as a toothache pain or throbbing pain, or like the ticking of a clock. With these symptoms, abscess may with confidence be diagnosed. An abscess may appear as a direct result of inflammation, but as often as not it is consecutive to some antecedent action, to some ostitis which had been treated and regarded as cured. It is, under these circumstances, due to the breaking down—caseation—of some old inflammatory products which nature's processes had failed to absorb or utilize; and it should therefore be regarded as a residual abscess in a bone, since it is analogous to such as are found in the soft parts, and particularly about joints.

Brodie, without doubt, was the first surgical author who, by his papers of 1845 (Lond. Med. Gaz., Dec. 12th, 1845, p. 1399) and 1846 (Med.-Chir. Transac., 1846), caught the ear of the profession of his time, and led his contemporaries as well as those who followed, to look upon such cases as a novelty, and the practice indicated as an innovation. So much so was this the case that Sir W. Ferguson, in 1864, in his lectures from this chair, described "the memorable instance in which Brodie amputated a leg for incurable pain in the tibia as one of the beacon lights of surgery never to be forgotten. It was, if I mistake not," he added, "the model case on which all our modern ideas about abscess of bone are founded, and the pathological examination of that limb led to a line of practice of inestimable value, which even at the present day (1864) is, I imagine, scarcely appreciated at its full worth." ("Lectures on Progress of Surgery," p. 35.) Yet on looking into the subject, William Broomfield, a surgeon to St. George's Hospital, where Brodie was educated, wrote in 1773: "Whenever a patient complains of a dull, heavy pain, deeply situated in the bone, possibly consequent to a violent blow received on the part some time before, and though, at the time the patient complains of this uneasiness within the bone, the integuments shall appear perfectly sound, and the bone itself not in the least injured, *we have great reason to suspect an abscess in the bone.*" ("Chirurgical Observations.") And John Hunter himself, who lectured on surgery at St. George's Hospital, when speaking of abscess in bone in 1787, said in one of his lectures: "The crown of the trephine is often necessary to be employed in order to get at the seat of abscess;" and he spoke as if the practice Brodie advocated later on was well recognized in his day—as, doubtless, it was. Brodie, at any rate, had forgotten it, and he did good in recalling the attention of surgeons to the subject. Brodie, however, went a step further than any other surgeon of his day, for he not only recognized the value of using the trephine when an abscess existed in bone, but he suggested the possibility of the practice being of use for the very purpose I am now advocating—the relief of tension; and he did so in the following words: "Even if abscess should not exist, I can conceive that the perforation of the bone, *by relieving tension and giving exit to serum collected in the cancellous structure, might be productive of benefit;* and at all events, the operation is simple, easily performed, and cannot itself be regarded as in any degree dangerous." (Brodie on "Joints," third edition, 1850, p. 298.) I am pleased, therefore, to be able to bring forward such a surgeon as Brodie to support me in the practice I am now advocating.

CASE XXXI. *Chronic Abscess in the Lower End of the Ulna, of Eight Years' Duration; Trephining; Removal of a small Sequestrum from the Abscess Cavity; Complete Recovery.*—Emma R——, aged twenty-five, a healthy married woman, came under my care in November, 1881, with an enlarge-

ment of the lower two inches of her right ulna, which had been
slowly coming for eight years. The affection had followed a
sprain. Pain, of a dull, aching character, had followed the
sprain and this had at times been felt up to the arm. When
seen, the bone in its lower two inches was at least twice its
normal size. The swelling was smooth, and to the touch painless; all the movements of the hand were natural. There
was a constant dull aching pain in the part, and at times the
pain was intense. The diagnosis made was that of chronic
inflammation. In December I cut down upon the bone, and
peeled back the periosteum, which was healthy. I then trephined the ulna, and found great difficulty in doing so on account of the density of the bone. Having removed a cylinder
of bone, I exposed a cavity about three quarters of an inch in
diameter, in which rested a small round sequestrum of bone,
surrounded with pus. The wall of the cavity was made up of
dense bone. After the operation all pain ceased, and a good
recovery followed. When seen by me five years later, the
hand and arm were as good as the other, except for the scar.

CASE XXXII. *Abscess in the Shaft of the Femur Simu-
lating a New Growth; Opening of Abscess; Cure.*—William
B——, a gardener, aged twenty, came up to me from Folkestone, by the advice of Messrs. Eastes of that place, for a swelling occupying the junction of the middle and lower thirds of
the left femur, which had been coming on, or at least had been
observed, for five months. For two years he had had pain off
and on in his left thigh, but he did not think there was any
swelling. Two months before being seen he had had an attack of bronchitis, and on his recovery from this the pain in
his left thigh became worse, and a swelling was discovered.
For two weeks he went about his work, although with pain,
which was not, however, very severe during the day, but at
night it prevented sleep. For two months he had been unable
to get about, and on account of this pain he sought advice.
When I saw him on January 6th, 1888, I found an ovoid
spindle-shaped enlargement of his left thigh-bone, extending
downward to the knee, and some effusion into the knee joint.
The swelling was very clearly defined, and on gentle manipulation was not painful; in certain parts, however, firm pressure was resented. The limb measured an inch and a quarter
more on the affected than on the sound side. The man went
into Guy's Hospital for treatment. Two days after I first saw
him a change had taken place in the tumor. It was less defined; the old pain had gone; but the swelling was tender.
There was likewise more swelling in the adjacent soft parts,
and also there was more heat. On January 13th the swelling
was explored through an incision made on the anterior and
outer part of the thigh, over the tender spot; and when the
bone was reached a small discharging orifice, just large enough

to admit a probe, communicating with the interior of the bone was found. From this orifice pus exuded. The abscess cavity in the bone was then laid open by means of a chisel and strong scalpel, and about two ounces of pus were evacuated. There was no necrosed bone found. The cavity in the bone was smooth. I well washed and syringed out this cavity with hot iodine water; with the same lotion thoroughly irrigated all the soft parts into which pus had escaped, and dressed the wound with iodoform gauze dipped in terebene oil, after having introduced a drainage-tube into the abscess cavity. The limb was then secured upon a back splint. In the subsequent history of the case there was nothing striking to relate, for recovery went on steadily and painlessly, and in two months the wound had healed. Later on the wound reopened, and some dead bone, which had formed the wall of the abscess, was removed.

Trephining a bone the seat of chronic ostitis, or of what is often called *condensing* ostitis, is an operation of recognized value, although it has, as a rule, been undertaken from a mistaken diagnosis, and under the belief that a chronic abscess in the bone existed. The experience thus gained has, however, taught surgeons an important lesson, and that relief to a prolonged, persistent, and disabling pain in a chronically inflamed bone may be expected to follow the operation of trephining. Under such circumstances it may well be a matter of surprise that the principle upon which the operation proved of value has not been more fully recognized, and that the expediency of relieving tension in a bone the seat of a chronic inflammation has not been accepted. For it might have been fairly argued that if in a chronically inflamed bone relief to pain may be expected to follow the operation of trephining, even when the disease has persisted for many years, the same operation, or its equivalent, if applied earlier, would not only bring about equally good results, but at the same time tend to prevent or modify the changes in the bone which are generally met with in such cases, and which the preparations in our museums so abundantly illustrate. That there is truth in this argument it is quite impossible for me to doubt; and I am convinced that if surgeons would, as a principle of practice, apply their art to relieve tension in all bones the seat of inflammation, much suffering would be saved and fewer bones and limbs sacrificed; the cases of inflammation of the bone would be far more amenable to treatment, and a principle of practice would be introduced which would bring these hitherto difficult cases of disease within the limits of curable affections, without the frightful destructive changes with which we are all too familiar. By way of illustration I append the brief notes of a few cases in which success followed treatment.

Case XXXIII. *Chronic Ostitis of the Shaft of the Tibia of Sixteen Years' Standing; Trephining; Cure.*—C. H——, aged twenty-nine, came under my care in January, 1885, with an enlargement of the shaft of the right tibia at the junction of the upper and middle thirds of the bone, which had been coming on for sixteen years, or more than half the man's life, and had followed a severe blow. The bone measured transversely at the spot indicated one inch more than its fellow, and vertically the swelling occupied about three inches of bone. To the hand the affected bone felt hotter than the other, but there was no pain on pressure. There had been during the past sixteen years a constant aching pain in the part, and after much exercise a throbbing. The pain was always worse at night. There was no history of syphilis, and the patient generally was fairly well. Having diagnosed chronic ostitis, I trephined the bone in the centre of the swelling, and used a large trephine. I perforated down to the medullary cavity, although with difficulty, as the bone was very dense. I also drilled the bone in two other directions from the trephine opening. The operation gave full, immediate, and permanent relief to all the symptoms, and a good recovery followed. I saw this gentleman a year later, when he was quite well, the bone having much contracted.

Case XXXIV. *Chronic Ostitis of the Shaft of the Tibia of Four Years' Duration; Trephining; Cure.*—Alice J——, aged sixteen, came under my care in December, 1878, with considerable enlargement of the upper third of the right tibia, thickening of the soft tissues over it, and pain of a severe character in the part. The pain, which was at times aggravated, was said to resemble the "ticking of a clock." Her temperature was 100°. The swelling had been slowly coming on for four years after a fall upon a stone. I cut down upon the part, and, having reflected some thickened periosteum, trephined the bone down to the medullary canal. The bone which was removed by the trephine was dense, like ivory. Everything went on well after the operation, and the original pain at once ceased. The wound granulated up in a month, and when seen six months later the patient was well. She had not had any return of pain, and the thickened bone was fining down. The temperature, which was 100° at the operation, fell to normal, where it remained.

Case XXXV. *Ostitis of the Shaft of the Tibia; Trephining of the Bone, with Relief to Pain; Subsequent Necrosis;*

Recovery.—James W——, aged twenty, came under my care in June, 1860, with enlargement of the shaft of his right tibia from inflammation following a blow eight months previously. The bone was much expanded, and the seat of a constant, and at times intense pain, which was always worse at night. I trephined the bone, and removed a central circular piece of bloodless, dense, waxy-looking bone and, as a result, all pain permanently ceased. Some limited necrosis, however, took place at a later period, and after the sequestrum was removed recovery followed.

CASE XXXVI. *Ostitis of the Lower Half of the Shaft of the Right Humerus; Drilling the Bone; Recovery.*—I was consulted by M. R——, a healthy-looking youth, aged seventeen, in September, 1871, for a considerable enlargement of the lower half of his right humerus, which had been steadily increasing for at least five years. It was the seat of a constant pain, which was always worse at night ; at times he had attacks of very severe pain in the part. He could give no history of injury. When I saw him the bone seemed to be uniformly enlarged and smooth. It was not painful on gentle manipulation, but firm pressure over the bone excited pain, as also did forcible movements of the joint. I looked upon the case as one of chronic ostitis, and drilled the bone at its outer aspect in three or four places. Blood alone escaped. All pain, however, left the part after the operation and the wound healed. Six months later the patient was well, and the bone had much diminished in size.

CASE XXXVII. *Chronic Ostitis of the Tibia of at least Ten Years' Duration; Trephining of Ivory-like Bone; discovery of a small Sequestrum in the Bone; Rapid Recovery.*—Mrs. M——, a lady of about thirty-five years of age, consulted me in July, 1880, with a tibia which was clearly much enlarged about its centre, and the seat of a dull aching pain for at least ten years. She was married, and had been much in India. She was apparently in other respects healthy. The pain in the bone was constant; but at times, and particularly at night, it was much worse. The bone where it was affected was about twice its normal size. There was no history of injury. I regarded the case as one of chronic ostitis, and accordingly trephined the bone, Dr. Wyman, of Putney, kindly assisting. I used a trephine about three quarters of an inch across, and never had so much difficulty in removing a cylinder of bone, that which was cut through being like ivory. Having cut well into the bone, I removed the cylinder and found at its base a small spiculum half an inch long, resting in a cavity which just fitted it. This sequestrum I removed. The operation at once gave relief, but the wound was some four months in healing. The pain the patient had endured, however, never returned. This lady is now quite well, and has never had any more trouble with, or pain in, her leg.

My colleagues have likewise followed the practice I am now inculcating. Thus, three cases of acute ostitis have been treated by drilling; and in all pus was evacuated. In one of these two cases recovery at once took place, and in the remaining the necrosis that followed was only superficial. Twelve cases of the drilling of bones for chronic ostitis have likewise taken place in the practice of other colleagues, and in each one relief to pain was at once afforded. In seven of these cases a speedy recovery followed the operation, although the symptoms of local ostitis had existed for years, varying from two up to twenty-six. In six of the cases there had been severe local pain from six to ten years. Four other cases were much relieved by the measure, but it is not known whether they were cured. In the twelfth case the hip disease for which the operation was undertaken was not arrested. The operation of trephining bone was performed on seventeen other occasions, and in thirteen of these speedy recovery was the result of the measure, although in one with subsequent necrosis. In three instances relief was given by the operation, but the joint disease for which it was undertaken, with the view to its arrest, continued, and had to be treated. With these hard facts, based on an analysis of thirty-two cases, it can hardly be said that the operation of drilling or trephining inflamed bone is not successful.

Time tells me that I must now draw to a conclusion; and as I have applied the principle of practice I am advocating to every variety of inflammation of bone, I may be allowed to summarize the whole in the following conclusions:

1. The pain associated with every form of inflammation of the bone or of its periosteal covering is due to tension, and the severity of the pain is a fair measure of its intensity.

2. In acute inflammation of the bone or its periosteum, tension is the chief cause of necrosis; and in the subacute and chronic forms it is a potent cause of their chronicity, as well as of the destructive changes which as a rule follow.

3. The relief of tension, wherever met with, when the result of inflammation, is an important principle of practice which should be always followed. In bone the principle is most imperative, on account of the difficulties under which natural processes act in that direction, by reason of the absence of

elasticity or yielding in bone, and by reason of the anatomical arrangements of its vessels which favor blood stasis.

4. To relieve tension in the softer tissues of the body, the local application of leeches, local or general venesection, acupuncture, aspiration, punctures, and incisions may be requisite; whereas, to carry out the same practice in endostitis or periostitis, subcutaneous or open incisions down to the bone, and the drilling, trephining, or laying open of bone by a saw, may be required, the choice of method having to be determined by the requirements of the individual case.

5. In the early or hyperæmic stage of inflammation of bone, before destructive changes have taken place, experience seems clearly to indicate that the relief of tension—as indicated by a dull aching pain, etc.—by means of drilling or trephining into bone, may arrest the progress of the disease, and help toward a cure by resolution; whereas, in the exceptional cases in which this good result does not take place, suffering is saved and destructive changes are limited.

6. In articular ostitis of every kind and variety and in every stage, this mode of treatment cannot be too strongly advocated, as tending toward the prevention of joint disease.

7. In acute or chronic abscess of bone, diaphyseal or epiphyseal, the abscess cavity must be opened, drained, and dressed in the most appropriate way—the principles of treatment being the same in hard or soft tissues, although they are modified by the anatomical conditions of the parts.

With these conclusions, Mr. President and gentlemen, I close my lecture. I fear much that to some I may have proved wearisome; and more, that I have failed to convince others of the value of the practical principle I have brought before you. My wish has been to carry conviction to every mind, and where I may have failed the fault must have been more in the way the subject has been placed before you than in the matter itself. At any rate, gentlemen, I have to thank you for your kind attention, and to express the hope that your own reflections on the subject will fill up my deficiencies, and that in the end all will be convinced that the relief of tension in inflammatory affections generally, if not always, is as a principle of practice worthy of adoption.

LECTURE III.

ON CRANIAL AND INTRACRANIAL INJURIES.

THE subject of tension, to which my two former lectures were devoted, leads in no unnatural way up to the consideration of cranial and intracranial injuries, for most, if not all, surgeons will be ready to admit that in such cases the evil effects of tension are notably manifested, and that operations undertaken with the object of evacuating either effused blood or inflammatory fluids pent up within a closed cavity such as the skull—that is, for the relief of tension—are of especial service. It is not my intention, however, to dwell at any length upon this aspect of the question, for I have thought it well to use my present opportunity to bring before you some general considerations on the subject of cranial injuries, which I have good reason to believe are neither sufficiently recognized nor generally taught, and more particularly since these considerations have no unimportant influence on surgical treatment.

As a preliminary reflection, I would emphasize a point which the surgeon should ever bear in mind in all head injuries—viz., that the effects of a force applied to the skull are much influenced by its thickness, and that in this matter there is in cranial bones great diversity. Under these circumstances, a slight blow on a thin skull may bring about a fracture, and no general cerebral injury, since the vibrations originated by the force of impact are expended locally upon the part struck, and are not carried along the bony basal ridges so as to vibrate in the brain structure and bring about mischief. Whereas, while a severe external force may fail to cause a fracture of a thick skull, it may start such intense vibrations within the cranium as to cause bruising or laceration of the brain, either of its surface or of its substance, at a point remote from the seat of impact, and even at times produce laceration of the venous sinuses or of the middle meningeal artery. In the former case the injury on the face of it looks severe; whereas it may be comparatively trivial, since there is no cerebral injury. In the latter instance the injury may appear slight, although in reality it is one which bodes death from cerebral mischief.

To say that injuries of the head should always be estimated *primarily* with reference to the amount of damage the cranial contents have sustained, and *secondarily* with reference to the risk of their becoming involved, is to say what all sound surgeons of experience believe and make the basis of their treatment. And yet students are taught to think that scalp wounds, fractures of the skull, hemorrhage beneath the bone, concussion and compression of the brain, and inflammation of the brain are separate and independent affections, with diagnostic symptoms which can be tabulated. The surgeon, however, who goes to the post-mortem room for information, knows too well that in every case of cranial injury of any importance there are certain brain changes common to most, if not all, which should be fully recognized and taken into account in its diagnosis, prognosis, or treatment; and that, should either a fracture, with or without depressed bone or intracranial hemorrhage, coexist in the same case, such a condition had better be regarded as a complication of the common factor rather than as one which stands alone. For example, a man falls or receives a blow upon the head, and is for a time "stunned" —that is, rendered more or less senseless from paralysis of brain function; he is said to be suffering from "concussion of the brain," whatever that term may mean. Another man, as a result of the same kind of accident, receives in addition to the "stunning" a scalp wound, with a fissure either in the vertex or base of his cranium; and he is described as one who is suffering from a compound fracture of the skull, either of the vertex, base, or of both. A third man comes under observation in the same state of so-called concussion, but with a depressed fracture of bone, complicated or not with a scalp wound, and as a result of this depression there may or may not be other symptoms, or those present may be intensified. Under either circumstance, however, his case is described as one of depressed fracture of the skull, giving rise to compression of the brain. Yet in all these different classes of cases there is one common injury, one common source of danger, present or remote—viz., the condition of the brain which is associated with the injury, and which has been brought about by the "stunning" force. If the general cerebral injury be trivial, the local complication of a scalp wound, or even of a fissured or depressed fracture, is, although serious, comparatively unimportant; if it be of a grave nature, the local complication must, however great, sink into insignificance.

What, then, it may be asked, is the condition of a brain in a state of so-called concussion? Let us inquire. Concussion of the brain means, in a physiological sense, a sudden and more or less complete arrest of the brain's mental and physical functions, brought about by external violence. The brain in its bony case has been made to vibrate more or less roughly either by some general shake of the whole frame, or by some local violence applied directly or conveyed indirectly to the cranium as a localized or diffused force, the effects of this force upon the brain being of necessity proportional to its concentration and intensity, and in a degree to the age and healthiness of the brain structure and the thickness of the cranial wall. Thus, a concentrated blow with a blunt or edged instrument, probably, and in a thin skull certainly, spends its force in producing a local cranial or cerebral injury; whereas, any force of a diffused nature, directly or indirectly applied, and whether causing a fracture of the cranium or not, more likely brings about some structural change in the cerebral tissue, remote from, rather than at, the seat of impact. And should the brain or its vessels, in either case, have undergone senile or any morbid change, it is more prone to suffer seriously from such external violence than a healthy organ. In every case, therefore, of injury to the head, the brain is made to vibrate more or less forcibly; when the vibrations are feeble, the injury to the brain structure resulting therefrom is but slight; when they are severe, the mischief may be great. The complication of a fissure or fracture of the skull does not of itself, of necessity, tend to aggravate the cerebral mischief; although its presence may be regarded as a measure of the force which has brought it about. In all cases of cranial injury, therefore, the conclusion is clear that the cerebral mischief is the common factor, and the one important point to be taken into account.

This conclusion subsequently leads to the important question, What are the changes found in the brain after so-called concussion of its substance, or rather shaking of its structure? What are the structural changes, if any, which can be made out on the post-mortem table? For, of course, an answer to these questions can only be given from the observation of cases which have proved fatal, either directly from the injury, or at some remote period after the injury from other causes. Happily, the answer to this question is neither difficult nor uncertain. For I may say that at Guy's Hospital for at least a quarter of a century there was no case of head injury examined—and such includes every case—in which there was not some coarse brain lesion found, readily visible to the naked eye; in which there was not some contusion of the brain surface, laceration of the brain either upon the surface or within its substance or more or less hemorrhage upon or into the brain. In fact, concussion, in a pathological sense, has been, in my experience, synonymous with contusion or laceration of the brain. Other surgeons have expressed the same opinion from this chair. Sir Prescott Hewett, thirty years ago, said: "In every case in which I have seen death occur shortly after, and in consequence of, an injury to the head, I have invariably found ample evidence of the damage done to the cranial contents." Mr. Hilton, who followed him, wrote: "We ought to consider a brain which has been subjected to concussion as a bruised brain." And Mr. Le Gros Clark, who lectured later, stated: "I have never made or witnessed a post-mortem after speedy death from a blow on the head where there was not palpable physical lesion of the brain." Neudorfer, of the Austrian army, declares that he has never seen concussion, as so-called, since in all cases he has examined cerebral injury was found to exist. And Fano, a celebrated French surgeon, has also come to the conclusion "that the symptoms generally attributed to concussion are due, not to the concussion itself, but to contusion of the brain or to extravasation of blood." In fact, all authorities now agree that, when death follows a severe shaking or concussion of the brain, contusion, bruising, or laceration of the brain is invariably present, and that when this is not found, the death is probably to be ascribed to some other than a cerebral cause; and I shall be able, later on, to show that when death does not take place as an early result of the damage, and the patient either dies of some other affection or of some remote consequence of the injury, the same evidence of cerebral contusion is generally present. When extravasation of blood upon or into the substance of the brain follows "concussion" or rather vibrating injury, it is to be explained in the same way—that is, by some injury done to the vessels of the brain itself, or to the venous sinuses within its membranes. When due to the bruising of the brain itself, the seat of injury is probably found on the side of the brain opposite to that of the cranium which received the blow; the bruising being brought about by what is rightly termed "contre-coup." A fall or blow upon the occiput is, as a rule, followed by some bruising of the anterior cerebral lobes; one upon the frontal region, by a bruising of the posterior parts of the brain; while lateral or vertical blows are felt more by the middle lobes. In severe vertical blows the base of the brain itself is bruised. The amount of extravasated blood depends upon the degree of force applied and the healthiness of the vessels in the injured part; diseased vessels easily giving way under a vibrating force to which the healthy would not yield. When the extravasation of blood is upon the surface of the brain, it is either within the cavity of the arachnoid or the meshes of the pia mater; and under each condition the blood gravitates to the base. When the extravasation of blood takes place into the structure of the brain, it may be found in any part of the cerebrum, cerebellum, pons Varolii, or even in the ventricles, the extravasation rarely showing itself in the form of one large clot, but commonly in small and numerous spots of extravasation, which cannot be wiped away, as if from small vessels.

Thus I found in one case of so-called concussion, in which the fatal result took place sixty hours after the injury from changes brought about by the severe shaking of the brain, unassociated with fracture, that the brain was bruised all over, and blood was effused at the injured spots; the fluid in the ventricles was blood-stained, and the ventricles themselves ecchymosed.

In another case of death from "concussion," without fracture, the result of a fall, in a man aged thirty-one, on the fifteenth day after the injury, in whom convulsions and coma supervened, a layer of blood was found universally diffused over both hemispheres, dipping between the convolutions, and passing downward toward the base. The clot, which was shreddy and of a dull reddish-black color, had evidently been effused for some days. The surface of the brain beneath the seat of injury was softened; and at the base, where it had been damaged by contre-coup, similar changes had taken place. The vessels were healthy.

In a third case, where death followed from "concussion," and the vessels were diseased, multiple extravasations were detected after death throughout the substance of the brain.

A fourth case was that of a man (C. K——), aged sixty-five, who came under my care with a scalp wound over the left half of the occipital bone and noisy delirium, having just previously fallen out of a truck on to his head. He had no paralysis or special head symptoms. The pupils were natural; the pulse was 70, and the temperature 99.2°. He became rational in twenty-four hours, but only remained so for a day, when noisy delirium returned, with refusal to take food. This condition lasted for fourteen days, when he sank, although food was regularly and carefully given by the œsophageal tube. After his death on the sixteenth day from the fall, the anterior lobes of the brain, with the fore parts of the middle lobes, were found much bruised and covered with extravasated blood.

And in a fifth case—that of a man aged thirty-five, who came to Guy's on March 31st, and died on April 1st, 1882, about fifteen hours after the accident—blood was found extravasated over the whole surface of the brain beneath the membranes, and the brain itself was much ecchymosed in fine points. The third and fourth ventricles were full of blood-clot. There was laceration of the fornix and right optic thalamus, and no other lesion. The man had fallen on his head when jumping off a van, and given himself a scalp wound, exposing the bone, to the left of the occipital protuberance. He walked into Guy's, and complained only of headache and a feeling of sickness. He refused to stay in the hospital, and left. Having walked 200 yards, he vomited, and his friends gave him a "small soda." He then vomited again, and being unable to stand he was brought back to Guy's, where he was admitted insensible and comatose, and died, as already stated, fifteen hours after his fall.

When fissured fractures of the cranium complicate brain

injuries, and these fractures are the result of some diffused force, the cerebral mischief is not likely to differ from that which has been just described, although, as the force to produce a fracture may presumably be greater than that which fails to do so, the intracranial injuries may be greater from the cerebral vibration. In some cases the brain itself may, in addition, be bruised at the seat of impact. On the other hand, where the force which produced the fracture is concentrated or the brain-case thin, there may be more of local brain injury at the seat of fracture, and less of distant mischief from brain vibration. And with the fracture there may be certain special complications, such as depression of bone with or without compression of the brain, injury to the dura mater, membranes, or brain from the fractured bone or external force, and extravasation of blood between the dura mater and the bone from rupture of the middle meningeal artery or some venous sinus. But all these are complications of, and additions to, the general injury. It must not be forgotten, however, that in exceptional cases a fracture of the skull may take place from a concentrated local violence without producing any cerebral disturbance, particularly over the frontal region.

To prove still more conclusively that "concussion" of the brain means bruising or laceration of the brain, with more or less hemorrhage, I propose to bring before you the particulars of some cases which have been examined at Guy's Hospital after death, at more or less remote periods after the receipt of the head injury; and which died from either an independent affection or some remote results of the injury. Such cases are not numerous, but they are valuable, at any rate, for my present purpose. I trust I shall not, therefore, prove wearisome in reading brief abstracts of some of them.

CASE I. *Cerebral Injury; Marked Evidence of Old Bruising of the Brain Found.*—A powerful middle-aged man was found by a policeman in the Borough Market sitting down in a fainting condition. The policeman gave the patient some brandy-and-water, and brought him to Guy's, where he soon became comatose and died. One of his friends said that he had received an injury to his head some weeks (?) previously. After death no external signs of injury could be made out, and there was no fracture of the skull. The anterior and middle lobes of the left hemisphere of the brain were adherent to the base of the skull. The base of the anterior lobe showed brown discoloration from old bruising, and the middle lobe was so firmly adherent to the bone that it tore away. "These changes," wrote Moxon, who made the examination, "could not have been less than several weeks old, probably at least three months." There was a large effusion of recent blood-clot (two ounces) over the right side of the brain. There was no blood in the brain, and no lesion of its membranes. The viscera were healthy.

CASE II. *Cerebral Injury Complicated with Fractured Base of Cranium Thirty-eight Days before Death; Bruising of the Brain.*—David E——, aged nineteen, came under my care on June 24th, 1874, having fallen off an omnibus on to his head. He was admitted into the hospital, partly unconscious, with profuse bleeding from his *left* ear, which lasted for two days, and was followed for another eight days by the escape of a clear fluid (cerebro-spinal). On the second day after the accident the facial nerve became paralyzed. The man died on the thirty-eighth day from broncho-pneumonia, having lost all his brain symptoms except the facial paralysis. On examination of the body, a fracture was found in the skull, across the petrous portion of the left temporal bone, from the turn of the lateral sinus groove behind into the middle fossa, laying open the tympanic cavity. There was no trace of repair in the fracture. The olfactory bulb on the *left* side was gone, and the brain about it was bruised. The central parts of the brain were soft.

CASE III. *Cerebral Injury Complicated with Fracture of the Base of the Skull Twelve Weeks before Death; Evidence of Bruised Brain.* (Preparation in Guy's Museum, 1084 [55].) —William B——, aged forty-six, came under the care of Dr. Hilton Fagge in 1873, with vomiting after food and pain over the pylorus, which proved to be due to abdominal cancer. He had been an epileptic for four years, and during that time had been growing darker. Five weeks before admission, after a fall on the head from a ladder, he became insensible for a brief period, and blood oozed from his *right* ear, mixed with some watery fluid, which continued to flow for two days. All head symptoms disappeared, although he occasionally lost himself during his illness. He died from abdominal cancer. After death, a fracture of the base of the skull, crossing the petrous portion of the right temporal bone, and running the whole length of the meatus auditorius externus, was found. The under surface of the two anterior lobes and of the points of the left middle lobe of the brain presented a tawny yellow discoloration, clearly the result of blood effusion at the time of the injury, and, as usual, it was more marked on the side opposite to that of the fracture. There was also a little superficial softening of the cineritious substance.

CASE IV. *Cerebral Injury Six Weeks before Death, Followed by Abscess.*—William D——, aged thirty, was admitted into Guy's with pleuro-pneumonia, in a condition which soon ended in death, in March, 1873. Six weeks before his admission a beam had fallen upon his head, hurting him, but not producing any marked head symptoms or any bleeding from the ears or nose. Indeed he had not given up work, but continued as an engineer's laborer for four weeks—that is, up to two weeks before admission, when he felt ill, shivered, and had severe headache; he also soon lost his taste for sweet things. When admitted he had no paralysis, only headache and drowsiness. His temperature was normal. He had no convulsions. After death the brain was found, on removal of the skull-cap, to be flattened, so that it appeared to have no convolutions. Its surface was discolored in parts from what proved to be abscesses. A large and rather old abscess had burst into the hinder part of the right lateral ventricle, filling it with pus.

Case V. *Cerebral Injury Complicated with Fractured Skull and Spine, etc.; Death Ninety-one Days Later.* (Preparation in Guy's Museum, 1084 [52].)—George G——, aged twenty-seven, came into Guy's Hospital, under the care of Mr. Forster, in July, 1882, having fallen or been thrown out of a third-floor window. He was conscious, and complained of pain in his back. He had a scalp wound over the occiput, and evidently a fracture of the occipital bone. His lower limbs were paralyzed from a fractured spine. The patient died of pleurisy. At the necropsy a fissure was found in the right half of the occipital bone, which extended vertically across the root of the petrous portion of the right temporal bone toward the lesser wing of the sphenoid. In the posterior cerebellar fossa there were two offsets, one of which ran down to the foramen magnum. There were but feeble signs of repair in the fracture. The brain at the right anterior lobe was much bruised. There was blood between the bone and the dura mater, and on the inside of the dura mater there was much brown pigment. The eleventh dorsal vertebra was fractured.

Case VI. *Cerebral Injury Six Months before Death, Brought about by Meningeal Apoplexy; Marked Evidence of Old Cerebral Injury.*—Patrick H——, aged forty-one, was admitted into Guy's Hospital, under Dr. Pavy, in March, 1874, in a comatose condition, and soon died. He had been drinking for some days before, and had had a fit. Six months before, or thereabouts, after a fall down some stone steps, he was brought into the accident ward with a bruise over the right mastoid process and discharge of blood from the right ear. He was partially insensible for ten days, and was stupid for some time after. His pulse ranged from 40 to 50. He left convalescent and returned to his work, at which he continued until he had the fit for which he was readmitted just before his death. At the necropsy no injury of the cranial bones could be discovered. The dura mater over both sides of the brain presented on its inner surface a tawny red color, apparently stained with old extravasated blood. That covering the left hemisphere was smooth, but that over the right was in part lined with adherent coagulum which in some parts was of a brownish color, in others black. Some of it was evidently old. This was part of a large mass of coagulum which lay between the dura mater and the brain, on this side flattening the brain. The surface of the brain was so discolored from staining with blood that the amount of clot was difficult of determination. The brain had evidently been deeply bruised at the time of injury at the inferior surface of both anterior lobes and the summit of the right middle lobe, particularly toward the back of the lateral surface of the right hemisphere, where there was an irregular fissure, with much tawny discoloration of the tissue. The lateral ventricles were healthy. The large effusion of blood clearly came from the rupture of the vessels of the softened part, and was probably in part due to alcoholic stimulants.

CASE VII. *Cerebral Injury Thirteen Months before Death; Marked Evidence of Brain Injury.*—George L——, aged twenty-two, was admitted into Guy's Hospital under Dr. Habershon in February, 1871, in a semi-torpid condition, having been found by a policeman in a fit after a day or more of drunkenness. He could be roused with difficulty, and when roused moved all his limbs. He had right facial paralysis. His pulse was 44; the pupils were contracted. He gradually sank. He had had a severe injury of his head thirteen months previously, from which it was supposed he had recovered. After death no signs of injury of the cranial bones were discovered. The brain was flattened, and the anterior and middle lobes were adherent to the dura mater at the base, and the brain tore away when an attempt was made to remove it. The membranes of the brain at the base were very thick, and partly opaque white, partly of an ochre-yellow color; this appearance was confined to the membranes. The aperture into the fourth from the third ventricle was closed by some recent, lymph, and the brain bordering the channel was soft. The lateral ventricles were greatly dilated, the descending cornu on the left side projecting like a blister at the base of the brain. The left middle lobe was diffluent.

CASE VIII. *Cerebral Injury Two Years before Death from Phthisis; Marked Evidence of Bruised Brain.*—Wm. C——, aged fifty, came into Guy's Hospital with phthisis, under the care of Dr. Moxon, in 1874, and died within a few days. He was a sailor, and had enjoyed good health up to two years previously, when he had a high fall, and was stunned and bled from his left ear. The next day hot fluid came from the ear. He was laid up for three weeks, and when he left his bed he was giddy for nearly one year. He returned to his work, although deaf in his left ear. Five weeks before, his admission

13

he "caught a cold and cough," and died of acute phthisis.   At the post-mortem examination no clear indication of fracture of the petrous portion of the left temporal bone could be made out, although there was a slight transverse line across the bone.   There was an old bruise of the anterior lobe of the brain on the left side and slightly of the base of the middle lobe. That on the anterior formed an irregular hollow the size of a shilling.   The gray substance was quite destroyed, and microscopically was found to present hæmatoidin crystals and compound granular masses.

CASE IX. *Cerebral Injury Complicated with Fracture of the Base of the Skull on the Right Side Eight Years before Admission, Followed by Fits, Chronic Hydrocephalus, Spinal Curvature, Emphysema, and Hydrothorax; Marked Evidence of Old Bruising of the Brain.* (Preparation in Guy's Hospital Museum, 1084[56].)—David W——, aged thirty, was healthy until eight years before admission, when he fell off a ladder and hurt his head. Since then he had not been able to do hard work, and his memory had failed him. Five years ago he had a fit, and others had followed. He was admitted under Dr. Wilks in 1876, in a fit, comatose, and passing urine under him; but he gradually recovered sensibility in a few days. In the hospital he had a fit, and both sides of his body were convulsed; when consciousness returned, it was found that the *left* side of his body had diminished sensation, but he said this had existed for eight years, and was gradually growing worse. He was fairly intelligent, and answered questions readily. His pulse was slow, 38 to 40. He died of bronchitis. At the necropsy the brain was found to be flaccid. At the base of the right middle fossa, and over the roof of the orbit, there was a layer of brown pigment; also in the posterior fossa. The same pigment existed in patches over the base of the brain. There were fourteen ounces of fluid in the ventricles. The brain substance was healthy. The foramen magnum was altered in shape, and narrowed antero-posteriorly, the transverse diameter being much larger than the other. There was fracture of the right side of the base of the skull. The spine was curved at the sixth dorsal vertebra toward the right. The cord was healthy. The lungs were emphysematous; fluid existed in the left chest.

CASE X. *Cerebral Injury Complicated with Fracture of the Skull Nine Years before Death; Evidence of Old as well as of Recent Brain Injury.*—Michael L——, aged fifty, came under Mr. Cock's care on December 29th, 1867, and died on January 7th, 1868. He had fallen twenty feet on to the side of his head, and was admitted with a scalp wound and depressed fracture of the left of the vertex. He was unconscious on admission, but not paralyzed, and was never clear enough to give a history of his accident. One of his friends stated that he had had an injury to his head nine years previously.

After death the cranial bones were found to be thin. On the occipital base, about the left part of the groove for the toreular Herophili, were *fine* rough elevations, and here the dura mater was very adherent. About this part there was an old depressed irregular fracture of the bone, the bone being now united to the rest. Within the skull there was an elevation corresponding to the external depression, and its edges were bevelled off. There was no sign of any old external wound over the fracture, or of blood between the bone and dura mater; but on opening the latter about an ounce of liquid clotted blood was found effused over the left vertex, corresponding to the recent scalp wound. The right anterior lobe of the brain was adherent over the orbit, and the brain here was discolored brownish-yellow, as from old hæmatoma, this part corresponding to the spot of contrecoup from a blow on the left back of the head.

CASE XI. *Cerebral Injury Complicated with Fracture; Evidence of Brain Bruising, Recent and Old.*—Michael W——, aged fifty-three, came into Guy's Hospital, under Mr. Cock, in February, 1867, and died in two days. He was found in the street insensible, with a wound on the back of his head and bleeding from both ears, but chiefly the left. He died comatose. At the necropsy there was clear evidence of a heavy blow having been given over the right mastoid process, the bone at this part being fractured. There was no blood between the bone and dura mater at this part, but there were about two ounces between the dura mater and the brain. There were *recent* contusions on the anterior and middle cerebral lobes, and *old* yellow discoloration of both middle lobes. The right one was firmly adherent to the middle fossa outside the foramen ovale. Lining the dura mater of the right middle fossa of the base of the skull there was a thin membrane, easily separable; and this was thickest where the brain was adherent. The right middle lobe was more deeply bruised than other parts, where it was fixed to the fossa.

CASE XII. *Compound Fracture of the Cranium, with Marked Brain Symptoms, Occurring Three Years and a Quarter Previously; Necrosis of the Inner Table of the Skull; Removal of the Bone by Trephining; Death from Phthisis; Evidence of Bruised Brain and Extravasation of Blood.*—Conrad H——, aged forty-five, came under my care in January, 1879, with a discharging sinus on the right side of the occipital protuberance, communicating with the interior of the cranium, which had been the result of a compound fracture of the skull he had sustained three and a quarter years previously. The injury was brought about by a blow from a large stone, which stunned him, and he remained unconscious for seventeen days. He was abroad at the time, and had no treatment. About one year afterward some pieces of necrosed bone were taken from a second fracture on the vertex of the

skull he had received at the same time. He had then some
slight weakness of his left side. For the last year the sinus
had discharged freely, and he had had much headache. Finding on examination that some necrosed bone could be felt
within the cranium in the direction of the internal occipital
protuberance, I trephined the bone with an inch trephine, and
enlarged the opening with Hoffmann's forceps. Having done
this, I removed numerous fragments of the inner table of the
skull, corresponding with the lateral and longitudinal sinuses.
The dura mater within was thickened, and covered with granulations. The operation gave much relief to his head symptoms; but his lung trouble slowly extended, and destroyed life
five months subsequently. After death the repair of the base
of the skull was found to be complete, but the bone was thick
and irregular. The opening in the cerebellar fossa was only
partially closed. The dura mater corresponding thereto was
thick. The torcular Herophili and sinuses were healthy. The
dura mater covering both cerebral hemispheres was tawny
with old extravasated blood; indeed, a thin membranous film
could be stripped off its inner surface. The summits of the
middle lobes of the brain at its base showed some tawny ero-
sion, evidently the result of former bruising. The lungs were
extensively diseased.

The evidence I have thus laid before you of the pathological
conditions of the brains of those who have suffered from what
has been so long known as "concussion of the brain" will, I
trust, be deemed sufficient to convince such as may be in doubt
that they are really examples of cerebral injury; that term
meaning cerebral bruising or laceration, with more or less
hemorrhage upon and into the substance of the brain or its
ventricles, the amount of injury of every kind varying in degree in each case. In some it may be very slight, and in
others severe.

You will likewise have probably observed—what the details
of the cases I have brought before you so forcibly demonstrate
—the lasting character of the changes which the brain may
have undergone as a result of injury, and the evident slowness
with which nature performs in this organ her reparative work;
for in some of the cases quoted, years· had passed after the
injury had been received, and yet marked evidence of its former
existence was still present. Indeed, such evidence as I have
laid before you of necessity draws out the question, Is a
bruised brain ever thoroughly repaired; and are not the
changes which the injury may have brought about fixed and

permanent? It is to be regretted that an answer to these
questions can only be given in an unfavorable form; and that,
while we may be hopeful as to this complete repair and recovery from a slight injury or bruise, we are bound to regard
graver cases in a more serious light, and to deal with them
accordingly, since what evidence we possess seems to show
that when any portion of the brain has been severely or mod-
erately bruised, it has been permanently injured. This evidence also dovetails in with the general experience, which tells
us not only of the presence of physical head symptoms, but
that the mental and moral characters of men are often permanently altered by a head injury.

With these facts and conclusions before us, am I, therefore,
wrong in assuming with some confidence that you will see
with me the expediency of combining with the term "concussion" that of "injury," and of describing such cases in the
future as those of injury of the brain from concussion? The
term "concussion" by itself is vague and delusive, while that
of "injury" is clear and true, and conveys at once a meaning
the force of which cannot be misunderstood. The word "concussion" later on may be dropped, and the simple term "injury" retained. With this starting-point, it would naturally
follow that fractures of the skull in all their varieties, hemorrhage into the cranium in all its forms, and compression of the
brain, however brought about, will be regarded as complications of the one common and essential factor, cerebral injury,
and not, as now, be regarded as separate and individual troubles
to be dealt with independently. And even scalp wounds, the
result of external violence, would assume a position in the surgeon's mind they ought to have, but have not yet attained;
and consequently receive the attention to which they are en-
titled, not so much perhaps on their own individual account
as simple wounds, but as wounds mostly brought about by
direct violence applied to the cranium, and consequently liable
to be complicated with some contusion of the cranial bone or
intracranial injury.

Up to this time my observations have been confined to the
elucidation of the first of the two main clinical points which
have had a common bearing upon all cranial injuries, and to
which I drew your attention at an early period of this lecture
—namely, "that all injuries of the head should be estimated

primarily with reference to the amount of damage the cranial
contents have sustained;" and I trust I have demonstrated
with sufficient clearness that a cerebral injury of some kind
is the one common factor.   I propose now, therefore, to pass
on and consider the treatment of cranial and intracranial injuries, and, with the light which the above conclusion throws
upon the whole subject, see what bearing it ought to have
upon the second clinical point to which attention has been
drawn—viz., "that injuries of the head should be estimated
secondarily with reference to the risk of the cranial contents
becoming involved;" and it should be remembered that this
risk is one to which every degree and variety of cranial injury
is liable.   In even such an apparently simple accident as a
contusion of the head, whether with or without a scalp wound,
the fear of this secondary danger ought not to be overlooked;
indeed, it ought always to be held in view, for I imagine there
are but few surgeons who have not been called upon to treat
examples of scalp wounds, or patients who, having had cranial
blows and being supposed to have been cured, have, on going
to work or moving about, or after some indiscretion of diet,
complained of headache, restlessness, giddiness, nausea, or
even vomiting, with more or less febrile disturbance—all these
symptoms being those of cerebral irritation, or the first step
of inflammation.   Or possibly the patient has complained
only of local pain at the seat of injury, and the surgeon on
examination finds some swelling of the soft parts over the
bone or some change in the appearance of the wound, its
healthy granulating surface having assumed a pale, flabby
condition, always suggestive of an early ostitis or periostitis.
"Acceleration or hardness of pulse," wrote Percival Pott,
" restlessness, anxiety, and any degree of fever, after a smart
blow on the head, are always to be suspected and attended to.
. . . When there is a wound, it will for a time have the
same appearance as a simple wound.   But after a few days
all these favorable appearances will vanish; the sore will lose
its florid complexion and granulated surface, and become pale,
glassy, and flabby; instead of good matter, it will discharge
only a thin discolored sanies, and the pericranium will separate from the bone.   The first appearance of alteration in the
wound immediately succeeds the febrile attack, and as the
febrile symptoms increase the sore becomes worse and worse.

. . . Through the whole time, from the first attack of fever to the last and fatal period, an attentive observer will remark the gradual alteration of the color of the bone, if it be bare. At first it will be found to be whiter and more dry than the natural one, and as the symptoms increase the bone inclines more and more to a kind of purulent hue or whitish color." These extracts I have taken from the works of Percival Pott, who first drew attention to this danger of bone inflammation as a result of cranial injury a century ago, but possibly made too much of it. He regarded it as the chief element of danger in all cases of contusion, scalp wound, or fracture, and not only trephined the skull when ostitis existed, but laid it down as a rule that "perforation of the skull is absolutely necessary in seven cases out of ten of simple undepressed fracture." The operation for trepanning was called for in these simple cases " to *prevent* the effects of inflammation, detachment, and suppuration of the dura mater, and consequently the collection of matter between it and the skull." From this over-estimate of the value and necessity of the operation of trephining in cases of fracture, and the comparative rarity of cases of abscess between the bone and dura mater as a direct result of contusion, surgeons have been prone to treat too lightly the risks of a secondary ostitis following bone injury, whether complicated or not with scalp wound or even with fracture, and consequently to neglect what was good in Pott's teaching. As a result, I feel sure that many lives are lost yearly, and that many narrow escapes from death occur. I have the notes of some fatal cases of the kind before me, which I have taken from the post-mortem records of Guy's Hospital. In four of these pyæmia was the immediate cause of death, and such a result was probably brought about by the inflammation of the venous channels of the diploë of the injured bone. I will not weary you by reading all the details of the cases, but will lay before you their chief points.

CASE XIII. *Scalp Wound; Ostitis; Necrosis; Pyæmia.*— T. G——, a man aged twenty-two, having fallen from a height, came into Guy's Hospital with a scalp wound and a compound fracture of his leg; he died from pyæmia. The scalp wound had apparently healed, and the man with his compound fracture seemed doing well in all ways, when on the tenth day headache and febrile disturbance appeared, followed by swelling in the seat of cranial injury, reopening of the wound, and suppuration of the parts covering the bone, from which the pericranium had loosened. Indications of pyæmia soon appeared, but no general head symptoms, and he died in two weeks. At the necropsy, the anterior half of the parietal bone beneath the scalp wound was of a whitish color, bare for a space of three by two inches, and apparently dead. The necrosis extended through the bone, and on the surface of the dura mater beneath the bone there was lymph with pus, as also on the arachnoid surface. The brain was healthy. There were pyæmic abscesses about the body.

CASE XIV. *Scalp Wound; Ostitis and Necrosis of the Injured Bone; Meningitis; Pyæmia.*—Eliza S——, aged forty, came into Guy's Hospital with a large scalp wound over the right parietal region, and exposed bone. The injury was the result of a fall off an omnibus, which for a few minutes stunned her. The next day she complained of headache, and on the fourth day it was incessant. On the ninth day sleeplessness and indications of fever appeared; the wound also became unhealthy. On the twenty-first day there were rigors, and on the twenty-fifth some hemiplegia on the left side, for which the operation of trephining of the right parietal bone was performed, and some fetid pus evacuated from beneath the bone. The dura mater beneath the bone was velvety. Convulsions soon came on, and death in a week. At the necropsy, the whole thickness of the right or injured parietal bone was found to be dead, and the dura mater beneath discolored. The surface of the brain corresponding to the dead bone was covered with pus. Pyæmic abscesses were present in the lungs and liver.

CASE XV. *Scalp Wound; Ostitis of the External Table, Fracture of the Inner Table; Pyæmia.*—Edw. N——, aged eighteen, having received a scalp wound to the right of the vertex of his skull from a falling bucket, came to Guy's Hospital without any head symptoms, and had his head dressed. The wound healed rapidly without pain or trouble in about ten days, when some local swelling appeared, followed in two days by fever and rigors. In this condition he was admitted into the hospital, where pain and swelling of the right elbow-joint appeared, and later on chest symptoms, which proved fatal three months after the primary accident. After death, the outer shell of the parietal bone beneath the scalp wound, to the extent of an inch and a half by one inch, was necrosed, but it had not been fractured. The inner surface of the corresponding area of bone was fractured, the fracture lying in the long axis of the oval necrosed piece. The fracture was a mere fissure, slightly starred, and its edges were perceptibly raised. A little stringy lymph hung about the bone. Over the dura mater corresponding to the fractured bone there was a yellowish patch of lymph. The brain was healthy. There were pyæmic abscesses in the lungs, liver, and elbow.

CASE XVI. *Scalp Wound; Exposed and Inflamed Bone; Death from Bronchitis.*—A man, aged twenty-three, having been jerked from the shaft of a cart, received a blow and a wound over his left temple which exposed the bone. There were no head symptoms. The wound was carefully dressed antiseptically, and for a week everything went on well. At the end of that time his temperature went up to 104.6°, and the glands of his neck commenced to enlarge. On the tenth day he had paralysis of the left facial nerve, and bronchitis set in, which quickly destroyed the patient, three weeks after the injury. At the post-mortem examination, two square inches of the left or injured temporal bone were exposed. The bone was dry and discolored, but there was no obvious necrosis. The diploë of the bone in the line of section of the calvaria on the left side was more vascular than that on the right side. The brain and dura mater were healthy. The bronchial tubes were filled with viscid mucus. The other organs were healthy

CASE XVII. *Scalp Wound; Necrosis of Bone; Abscess in the Brain.*—A male child, aged three, six weeks before death fell on his forehead, causing a wound one inch above the left orbit. No head symptoms were induced by the fall, and for three days all seemed to be well, when he fainted in his mother's arms. He was then brought to Guy's Hospital, and requested to be left; but to this the mother objected. A few days later the child again fainted and vomited, and as the vomiting persisted the mother brought her child into the hospital. At that time, sixteen days after the accident, the wound had healed, and the scar was adherent to the bone. The child vomited daily, and his temperature was just above normal. A week later, without any important change in the symptoms, the child had a fit which lasted an hour. During the fit the right leg was rigid, and the arm with the fingers and thumb became spasmodically flexed. The left limbs also moved spasmodically. Temperature, 106°. In two days the child died. After death the frontal bone at the seat of injury was covered with purulent lymph beneath the pericranium. Beneath this the bone was rough and ulcerated. The inner table over a space the size of a sixpence was opaque yellow. When sawn through, a piece of the outer table was loose and necrosed. The dura mater at this spot was adherent to the brain. There was a little pus on its outer surface. The left frontal lobe of the brain beneath this spot was soft, swollen, and fluctuating, and when cut into was found to contain a large abscess of the size of an apricot, which had a distinct lining membrane. There was no red softening.

CASE XVIII. *Scalp Wound; Necrosis of Bone; Abscess of the Brain.*—A middle-aged woman three weeks before her admission into Guy's Hospital received a scalp wound from a blow upon the forehead. She continued at her work for two weeks, and it is said without any head symptoms, when she became comatose and died in a week. She was brought to the hospital in the dying comatose stage. At the post-mortem examination a sloughing wound was found to occupy the centre of her forehead, and beneath it bone was exposed. The surface of the bone was yellow and dead, but not depressed. The area of dead bone was separated from the living by a shallow groove. The inner surface of the bone was blackish; the diploë was full of pus. There was chocolate-colored pus beneath the dura mater of the injured part, and the brain beneath was suppurating, the abscess burrowing backward.

CASE XIX. *Contusion of Cranium; Pott's "Puffy" Tumor; Trephining; Meningitis; Death; Bruised Brain.*—W. L——, aged forty-six, was admitted into Guy's Hospital, under the care of Mr. Howse, on December 13th, 1882, fifteen days after having been knocked down by a cab and stunned. He was taken home after the accident, unconscious, and remained in that state for three hours. He then vomited and brought up blood. The next day he became drowsy; and four days later he had a convulsion, which was followed by others for three days. He then became delirious and unconscious. When admitted he was in a low typhoid state, constantly muttering and picking at the bed-clothes. Temperature, 100.4°. There was no paralysis. A swelling was found over the vertex of the skull. This was cut down upon, and blood was seen effused beneath the pericranium, which readily peeled off the bone. The bone was bruised and yellowish. The inch trephine was used. The dura mater, which bulged into the opening and was covered with lymph, pulsated. Nothing more was done, except that the wound was dressed and cold applied to the head. The delirium, however, continued, and gangrenous pneumonia set in, which proved fatal on January 13th, thirty days after the accident. After death the base of the brain was found to be bruised by contre-coup, and there was diffused meningitis.

The cases I have quoted were all examples of ostitis and necrosis, the result of a contusion of the bone associated with scalp wound. I could give as many more associated with fracture if they were needed, and they would all tell the same tale. In none of the cases were there any symptoms of brain injury after the accident, and in most the symptoms did not appear for a week or ten days or a fortnight afterward. In all, the mischief which produced death had clearly originated in the bone. In none of the cases had much care been employed to guard against the secondary mischief which took place, and which led on to a fatal issue; and it may reasonably be thought that, if judicious treatment had been applied from the receipt of the accident, no such result would have been recorded. The conclusion is therefore clear, that all scalp wounds which lead down to bone should be dealt with, for at least a fortnight or three weeks, with much care; and that such cases should, if possible, be treated as in- and not out-patients of hospitals for that time. For it is not the wound treatment only which calls for care, but the patient should be kept quiet, and given a simple unstimulating diet. Stimulants of all kinds should be forbidden, and meat allowed in very limited quantities. If at the end of two or three weeks, or thereabouts, no local or general symptoms appear to suggest mischief, the duties of life may be gradually recommenced. But even then a caution should always be given to observe care.

When local symptoms appear, such as have been described, a free incision down to the bone where no wound exists, or a free separation of the pericranium where there is a scalp wound, always does good. And should any symptom appear or persist which even suggests any intracranial complication, the operation of trephining should at once be had recourse to. "The spontaneous separation of the pericranium, if attended with general disorder of the patient, with chilliness, horripilation, languor, and some degree of fever, appears to me," says Pott, "from all the observations I have been capable of making, to be so sure and certain an indication of mischief underneath, either present or impending, that I shall never hesitate about perforating the bone in such circumstances. . . . When there is just reason for supposing matter to be found under the skull the operation of perforation cannot be performed too soon; it seldom happens that it is done soon enough. The perforation sets the dura mater free from pressure, and gives vent to collected matter, but nothing more. The inflamed state of the parts under the skull, and all the necessary consequences of such inflammation, call for all our attention fully as much afterward as before; and although the patient must have perished without the use of the trephine, yet the merely having used it will not preserve him without every other care." The prevention of this fatal trouble is, however, the more important point to emphasize; and for that purpose I bring the subject before you. Its early treatment may be beneficial and successful; its later treatment cannot be said to be so. Let us, therefore, teach the necessity of keeping patients with all but minor scalp wounds, and with those even where the bone is exposed, quiet and unstimulated for some weeks after the receipt of the injury where it can be done, and by so doing give nature an opportunity of repairing the mischief in the bone, which, though unseen, may reasonably be expected to be present after the application of a force sufficient to produce a scalp wound or a more severe injury. When a blow upon the head is known to have produced a fracture, the case is likely to be treated carefully; whereas, when no such fracture can be made out, and there is little or no external evidence of injury, the same care is not likely to be observed, although in both cases the violence which had been employed may have been equal. Yet in both cases the dangers of cranial ostitis from contusion are about the same. The fact, I am sure, requires to be emphasized, that cranial contusions, whether associated or not with fractures or with wounds, are always matters of serious importance, and as such should be treated from the first. Having dwelt upon the dangers of these cases, and illustrated some fatal results, I propose to quote a few examples of their successful treatment.

CASE XX. *Scalp Wound, and Subsequent Ostitis, Treatea by Trephining; Fissured Bone Discovered; Cure.*—Catherine S——, aged twenty-eight, came into Guy's Hospital in July, 1884, under Mr. Howse, with a scalp wound and fissured fracture of the skull, the result of a blow from a machine. She had no head symptoms, either at the time of the accident or after, and in six weeks she was discharged, supposed to be cured. A month later she was readmitted for continual headache and local pain in the seat of the former injury. She stated that she had not been able to work since she left the hospital. The old wound had reopened a week after leaving. On her readmission bare bone was felt—indeed, a piece of dead bone was taken away. In a day or so the pain in the head had much increased, even to make the patient scream. A crucial incision was then made down to the skull, when a fissured fracture was discovered. This operation did not give relief; consequently, she was trephined over the seat of fracture. The bone was found to be very dense and thickened, and its outer surface rough and pitted. No diploë existed. The dura mater was rough, and shaggy from adherent lymph. All cerebral symptoms had disappeared on the second day after the operation, and a rapid cure took place.

Case XXI. *Contusion of the Head; Ostitis; Trephining; Discovery of Fissured Fracture; Cure.*—Harry D——, aged five, was admitted into Guy's Hospital, under the care of Mr. Howse, on September 29th, 1880, having two weeks previously, in a fall, struck the left side of his head against a curbstone. He was unconscious after the accident for a few minutes, when he vomited. He was kept in bed for two or three days, and was supposed to be convalescent, when he had headache, and at night some lightheadedness. And these symptoms persisted up to his admission to the hospital. At this time, a fortnight after the injury, a fluctuating swelling about an inch in diameter was discovered beneath the seat of injury behind the coronal suture. There was some fever with night delirium, but no paralysis. He was trephined at the seat of swelling, when a fissure in the bone was discovered, and the dura mater was seen covered with lymph. From this time everything went well; headache and delirium disappeared, and convalescence followed.

Case XXII. *Scalp Wound; " Puffy " Swelling; Trephining; Cure.*—William T——, aged four, was admitted into Guy's Hospital, under Mr. Howse, on June 5th, 1885, having a week previously been struck above the right orbit by a swing, and received a scalp wound down to the bone. He progressed well for two or three days, when the wound began to inflame and he became feverish. In this condition he was admitted. The wound at this time was sloughing, and the bone was exposed. Temperature, 101°. A few days later, as no improvement took place, and the child was drowsy, the bone was trephined at a spot near the wound, which had become " puffy." The dura mater, where exposed, was granular, and the bone eroded. All symptoms at once disappeared, and a rapid recovery followed.

I will now pass on to consider the treatment of head injuries in the light of the view I am now advocating, for I am under a strong impression that such a view cannot do otherwise than have an important influence in rendering treatment more simple and intelligible; since, if in every grave, or indeed apparently uncomplicated example, associated with more or less complete paralysis of at least one of the brain functions, such as is indicated by unconsciousness, the surgeon recognizes to the full the force of the fact that the brain as a material organ is bruised or otherwise injured, a line of treatment is likely to be at once suggested which can best favor the restoration of the injured part toward health. Among the means which would probably find favor, physiological and mechanical rest would stand foremost, with the administration of nourishment simple enough to maintain the normal powers and help repair, and not stimulating enough to excite action. Everything in the form of alcoholic stimulants or solid meats would be forbidden; and this line of treatment would, moreover, be maintained for weeks, and possibly for months, the severity of the injury and the primary symptoms forming the surgeon's best guide to a decision. This careful line of treatment would also be adopted under the wholesome dread of exciting, by sins either of omission or of commission, the one common complication which the surgeon should ever have before him—namely, an inflammatory action in the injured organ. For experience speaks in no feeble terms that this action is readily started and with difficulty quelled, and that it is by such inflammatory changes in the injured brain that most head cases, simple or severe, are brought to a fatal termination. Mr. Hilton recognized this necessity nearly thirty years ago, for he taught "that recognized lesions of the brain and its membranes, associated with blows upon the head (whether the cranium be fractured or not), do not generally, or as a principle of treatment, obtain that extent of mechanical rest which is consistent with the expectation of perfect and complete structural repair. This error in the treatment of such cases is one of the chief sources of the diseases of the brain and its membranes which are met with in practice. . . . In cases of injury of what may be called the coarser structures, with more simple functions attached to them, we see that without perfect restoration of the structures their functions are not efficiently performed, and if used too early and too much they become painful and assume a chronic inflammatory condition. Such soft parts require weeks or months for their repair. Surely, then, we ought not to deny the necessary and proportionately much longer time for the repair of the more delicate brain tissues; a repair, be it remembered, which cannot be accomplished by any direct aid from the surgeon, but only by Nature herself employing her chief agent—Rest." It is a pleasure to me to be able to quote these apt sentences, framed by a former teacher and colleague upon this important subject—although many years have passed since they were uttered—to support the views it has been my privilege to bring before you—views, I may say, that I have for long taught at Guy's, and have reason to believe with some advantage.

Should symptoms of intracranial irritation or inflammation show themselves, they should be dealt with actively, as, from the nature of the brain and its membranous coverings, the process once started soon spreads. In the early stage the application of cold to the head by means of a Leiter's metallic tube is the most efficient local, and free purgation the most effective general, means, with very low diet. If the inflammatory action is great, a free bleeding from the jugular vein or from the arm is strongly to be advocated, and this operation may in many cases be repeated with much advantage. I am convinced I have saved some lives by this treatment. In chronic cases the value of mercury taken internally cannot be doubted.

These, then, are the common lines upon which the treatment of the common factor of all cranial injuries, simple or severe cerebral injury, should always be based; and they should likewise form the lines of treatment of all its complications. Thus, if a simple fracture of the vertex, base, or of both, complicates the case, the treatment is the same. The cerebral injury needs the surgeon's care, and not the fracture, which will take care of itself. A cranial fracture will heal in the same way as other fractures, but it will take a much longer period; and fractures of the base of the skull are apparently among the slowest. In specimens 1084[52] (eighty-four days), 1084[55] (ninety-one days), and 1084[56] (eight years), of the Guy's Museum, and in others of our own College museum, this point is indicated. The fractures of the skull will, at any rate, probably heal sooner than the cerebral injury will be repaired. The treatment for the latter will consequently have to be continued after the fracture has healed. If the fracture be but *slightly depressed,* whether simple or compound, and it appears only as a *fissure,* the case had probably better primarily be left alone, and dealt with secondarily on the smallest indication of cerebral trouble; for in these cases there is rarely comminution of the inner table, and consequently nothing in the form of bony spicules to fret and irritate the dura mater, and thus help forward a meningitis. To trephine in order to elevate this form of fissured fracture would therefore be to add another danger to a case in which the form of cerebral injury common to all already exists. If the fracture be *depressed, starred, or comminuted,* whether

simple or compound, the elevation of the depressed bone
should be the rule of practice, and the removal of all the
splintered fragments of the inner table carefully carried out,
the object of the operation being more to take away what, if
left, must irritate the dura mater, and so add to the existing
harm, than to relieve the depression. This operation should
be performed as much in simple as in compound fractures, for
the condition of the bones is the same in both; and with our
modern treatment of wounds the danger of the operation in
simple fracture is not materially increased. In *punctured
fractures* the operation of trephining, undertaken with the
object of removing the broken and displaced fragments of
bone, should be a rule of practice never to be deviated from.
The depressed and comminuted inner plates of bone to a certainty, if left, at a late if not early period of the case, irritate
the brain and its coverings, and so set up an encephalitis.

How far the presence or absence of what are called brain
symptoms should influence a surgeon in his decision as to
surgical interference in the different forms of depressed fractures of the skull we have been considering has been much
argued. For the surgeon is quite unable in bad cases of cranial injury to differentiate symptoms, and to say how far those
that are present in any individual case are due to the common
factor—cerebral injury—which resulted from the force that
produced the fracture, or how far they are caused by the depressed and fractured bone. But I am not sure that this is a
point of much practical importance, for in a bad case of fracture of the skull cerebral injury is probably already severe,
and the operation of elevating depressed bone and of removing
comminuted fragments is not likely to aggravate the trouble;
whereas in a less severe example in which the cerebral injury
is likely to be less serious, the existence of depressed bone and
of comminuted fragments must act injuriously, and should
consequently be removed. Under all circumstances, it is consequently the surgeon's duty to remove whatever sources of
trouble the presence of a depressed fracture may bring to an
already serious case of cerebral injury.

The operation of trephining or of elevation of bone in depressed fracture is called for more with the object of removing
from the brain what may or will be sources of local irritation
rather than with any view of removing the effects of the de-

pressed bone; for it is well recognized that, *per se*, a large area, and a considerable amount, of depressed bone are required to bring about symptoms of compression in an otherwise uninjured brain. Again, it is well known that a considerable extravasation of blood upon the surface of the brain, probably five or six ounces, whether between the bone and dura mater or in the cavity of the arachnoid, is required to bring about marked evidence of its presence, in the form of paralysis from compression. The rupture of the middle meningeal artery is a special complication of cranial injuries, or of fracture of the skull, but I do not propose to discuss it here at any length. I cannot, however, pass it by without referring to the exceedingly able article upon the subject published in the "Guy's Hospital Reports" for 1886, vol. xliii., p. 147, by my friend and colleague, Mr. H. A. Jacobson, since it contains not only a masterly account of every case on record up to date, but also a summary of the whole subject, which claims the close attention of every surgeon. His summary is as follows:

1. That the violence which causes middle meningeal hemorrhage is often slight, and that in these cases no fracture may be present.

2. That where there is a fracture, it is often a mere fissure, and may involve the internal table only.

3. That the history of the case, and, above, all, an interval of lucidity or consciousness, are invaluable, the latter being worth all the other symptoms put together.

4. That the symptoms of compression are in some cases deferred; that their onset may be then very sudden and rapidly fatal, failure of breathing being a marked feature.

5. That in those cases where the history is deficient, especially as to any interval of lucidity, and where it is difficult to be certain about the existence of hemiplegia, dilatation of the pupil on one side, that side corresponding to the clot, is a sign of great value. The explanation of this sign, that the third nerve is being pressed upon by a clot large enough to reach into the middle fossa, we owe to Mr. Hutchinson, with whose name in future this condition of the pupil should be associated.

6. That after trephining, exposure and partial removal of the clot, very severe hemorrhage may set in and prove difficult to arrest.

14

7. That in severer cases laceration or contusion of the brain are only too frequently complications.

This latter conclusion consequently links this special class of cases with the more general number of cranial injuries, and enables the surgeon to look upon them as a whole in the light in which I have now placed them before you.

There are many other questions in the surgery of cranial injuries which require elucidation, but time will not allow me to bring them under your notice. The points and questions I have selected are such as I believe to be most important to enable the younger surgeons and practitioners to read rightly the manifold and somewhat puzzling phenomena which severe cranial or cerebral injuries exhibit, and I have some confidence in the belief that, if the views I have expounded were accepted, the teaching and understanding of cranial or cerebral injuries would be greatly simplified. In conclusion, I must ask you who have listened to me so patiently and kindly to think over the questions I have ventilated, and to accept from me my warmest acknowledgments of the honor you have conferred upon me by allowing me, as your Hunterian Professor of Surgery, to deliver these lectures from this chair.

ANTISEPSIS

AND

ITS RELATION TO BACTERIOLOGY.

BY

DR. J. NEUDORFER,

Royal Staff-Physician and Director of the General Poliklinic, Vienna.

ANTISEPSIS

AND ITS RELATION TO BACTERIOLOGY.

"Nothing is lasting except Change, nothing is permanent except Mutation, nothing is settled except the Past,"—in these words does a gifted writer characterize politics; the same antitheses, in my belief, are applicable to medicine and to surgery, for in these sciences the beliefs of individuals are constantly changing, as well as the opinions of physicians in general, in regard to the most important questions. This change in belief occasionally occurs without attracting the special attention of some men, and they think that they stand on the same foundation, without noting the fact of its alteration, sometimes to the advantage and again sometimes to the disadvantage of truth.

Even as travellers on the deep, wide ocean take no account of the quiet, steady motion of the vessel, and notice it only when they reach their haven, and even as, further, they know not the direction of the port they have left nor of that to which they are tending—this knowledge being possessed by the officers and steersman alone from consultation of the charts and compass—even so does the practitioner make his way along the broad ocean of his daily life and occupation. Owing to his anxious and difficult daily task his attention may not be directed to the slow, but continuous progress in his science; he may not note the ever-changing phases of this progress; he only sees the change of scene after it has shifted, when he is conscious of the alteration of theory, method and practice of another. On this new basis he may stand for a decennium, until progress has again effected an alteration in the beliefs of medical science. He, however, who lives only in the past and looks not to the future, cannot have a complete understanding of that past. His thoughts and hands work empirically and by routine, and this is incompatible with quick alteration, and in so far progress is checked. It is advisable then to stop occasionally in order to consider the course of events in the past and the probability for the future. Thus we can see the generic relationship of the different stages of our art, and take account of the errors of the way which has been traversed.

Owing to the great and with difficulty circumscribed extent of the medical sciences, this backward and forward glance can only be taken in regard to established and limited questions, and I invite your attention to an *exposé* of the present state and future aspect of the antiseptic question.

Inflammation and Fever the Cardinal Symptoms of most Diseases since the Year 1800.

Even in olden times observers noted that the majority of internal and external diseases presented a constant chain of symptoms, such as swelling, redness, heat and pain in the affected parts, tissues or organs. In addition to these characteristic symptoms, there appeared at times an increase of the pulse rate and a general sense of ill-being of the patient.

These observations constituted then as now the character·istics of inflammation and fever. That tissue was said to be inflamed which was red, swollen, hot, painful; while in a patient in whom there existed an increase of the pulse rate, an elevation of the body and blood heat, and a change in the excreta and in the secreta, there was said to be fever.

Very often the causal connection between the inflammation and the fever could not be determined; often, again, the inflammation was not accompanied by fever, even as in many febrile states it was not possible to detect the inflammatory cause. As for the cause of the inflammation and the fever there existed no clear knowledge; only with the introduction of the microscope into medical research has it been possible to study experimentally the intimate sources of fever and of inflammation.

When the finger-web or the tongue, or, better still, the

mesentery of the frog (Cohnheim) is spread under the microscope, we see first a dilatation of the capillary net-work and a slowing of the blood stream. The white blood corpuscles move slowly along the vessel wall, while the red corpuscles remain in the centre of the vessel. The white corpuscles cling to the intima of the vessel, pass through the wall and then extravasate into the cellular tissue. · Soon after their movements cease, there occurs a momentary retrogression and then a stoppage of the circulation in the dilated capillary. Shortly after, the white corpuscles lose their pale-gray and homogeneous appearance and break up into sharply demarcated granules. As the inflammation increases there occurs a cloudiness due to the accumulation of white corpuscles which have passed through the vessel wall, and this renders further study by the microscope impossible. We can then only watch certain phases of the inflammatory process and we must judge hypothetically of the relation between the different phases.

As the inflammation progresses we find the white corpuscles in such great number that we cannot believe that they have come exclusively by migration. We believe, therefore, that a part have appeared from division of the leucocytes which have migrated from the vessel, and a part from prolifcration of the pre-existing cellular tissue cells. This phase of the inflammatory process is known under the name of suppuration. We no longer call the bodies in the fluid leucocytes, although they resemble these perfectly, but pus corpuscles.

In a still later stage of the inflammatory process we note the development of capillary vessels. This phase is called the granulation period. As to the other stages of the process— the formation of a so-called pyogenic membrane, the occurrence of phlegmonous inflammation, the period of cicatrization, etc., —we will not dwell on them, since they do not directly interest us.

We are certain of the following facts in regard to the progress of the inflammation: As well from experiments on animals as from study in man, we know that it consists in a dilatation of the capillaries, a migration of the leucocytes through the walls of the vessels, in a spreading and an increase of these leucocytes into the surrounding tissue, in a blood stasis in the dilated capillaries, in an increase of the blood stream, and a congestion in the immediate neighborhood of the inflammatory area.   These local changes are occasionally accompanied by general disturbances of nutrition and by fever.

These alterations, deduced from experiment and observation, accord entirely with the signs of inflammation laid down by Celsius, and which he termed *tumor, rubor, calor, dolor, atque functio læsa.*

MECHANICAL, THERMIC AND CHEMICAL IRRITATION AS CAUSES OF DISEASE.

The next question is in regard to the causes of the above changes in the inflammatory area and in the organism, for in the material world change without cause is not to be thought of.

From the earliest times it was assumed that an irritation was at the bottom of the changes to be observed in inflammation.   Mechanical, thermic, and chemical irritations were said to affect the tissues and the organs, altering the customary processes in them and causing an inflammation.   When the irritant affected the entire organism or spread throughout it then there occurred fever.   It was claimed, then, that mechanical injuries, burns or refrigeration (thermic irritation), cauterization with strong acid, alkalies, or mineral substances (chemical irritation), might cause inflammation and suppuration, and, often enough, fever.

In the present century it was supposed that, in addition to mechanical, thermic and chemical irritants, there were others to which I will apply the term organic, and that these also might cause inflammation, suppuration and fever.   Otto Weber and Theodore Billroth are to be named as early observers in this direction.   They came to the conclusion from their experiments that the above phenomena would result from the entrance into the animal experimented upon of very small amounts of organic substances.   They claimed that in blood, in pus, in tissue, by disintegration and chemical process, organic substances were formed which, when introduced into the blood in small amount, would cause inflammation and fever. These newly-formed organic substances, which they did not exactly isolate, they called phlogogenous and pyrogenous ferments.

A few years before (1856), Panum had determined that inflammation of the intestines of animals which had been poisoned by decomposed material, was due to a chemical substance which could not be destroyed by heat.

Later still, Bergmann and Schmiedeberg isolated from fecal matter a crystalline substance to which they gave the name of sepsin, and they determined that, when this was introduced into the bodies of animals, it caused exactly analogous symptoms to those which we find in septicæmia; still the observations of Panum, as well as those of Bergmann and Schmiedeberg remained without influence on medical and surgical practice.

A Contagium Vivum as the Cause of Disease.

Pasteur's observations first resulted in facts of value, especially from a surgical stand-point. Pasteur first claimed that the process of fermentation, of suppuration and of decomposition, as also the occurrence of contagious diseases, was due to the presence of an organized living cause, which he termed contagium animatum. He proved that the above processes might be forestalled by preventing the access of the microbe.

Pasteur, however, was not the original and only observer who taught the presence of a contagium animatum. We may trace this view back to the year 1700. Then the question was discussed under the term spontaneous generation, although this assumption is not related to contagium animatum, for, if we grant that a coccus or bacterium may develop of itself and need not be brought from outside into the body of an animal, then does the groundwork of bacteriology fall to the ground like a house built of cards.

Without detailing the views of Reddi or entering into the dispute between Buffon and Spallanzani, we will mention here only the following points:

Caignard de la Tour, 1836, determined that the torulla cerevisiæ was a microscopic vegetable cell which, through increase in its cells, broke up sugar into alcohol and carbonic acid, and that the fermentation ended in a sugar-containing fluid. With the death of the yeast cell, or when this through any cause could increase no longer, the fermentation and breaking up of the sugar stopped at once.

In 1837 Schwan determined that meat and other albumin-containing substances became decomposed by germs residing in the air. These germs developed at the expense of the albumin, and thus led to its decomposition. Although the views of Caignard de la Tour and of Schwan were tested and confirmed by many learned observers, they obtained no general recognition and remained the property of a few skilled experimenters. The great discoveries of Pasteur first convinced the world of the presence of a contagium animatum.

Pasteur's methods of observation and of experiment are to-day above criticism on account of their precision, exactness and clearly established premises. The fortunate application of his theoretical conclusions to practical and material questions of to-day, has enabled Pasteur to prevent the periodical appearance of the phylloxera and to suggest prophylactic means against and to cure the effects of certain animal parasitic diseases. He has thus saved to France an annual loss of a hundred million francs. Further, physicians, physiologists, pathologists, botanists, hygienists, have studied and experimented in a similar direction in order to apply these theoretical considerations for the benefit of mankind. The result is that the literature of this subject has become enormous. Yet more, bacteriology has become the basis of the medical sciences, and the question in regard to which there is most dispute among physicians.

THE CONTAGIUM VIVUM IN SURGERY.

Here, in the fore-rank, a man must be named who applied Pasteur's observations in regard to the contagium vivum to the practice of surgery.

Joseph Lister, noticing the favorable progress of subcutaneous wounds in comparison with the unfavorable of open wounds, claimed that this difference was due to the micro-organisms from the air which, reaching the secretion of open wounds, there developed and increased and caused suppuration and infection; while, in case of subcutaneous wounds, the epidermis prevented the entrance of micro-organisms, and protected the extravasation and the exudation at the wound-site from infection.

Lister first, in 1867, seeing that he could not prevent the

access of micro-organisms to the open wound, began by killing them or rendering them incapable of development by means of carbolic acid.

In the Lancet for July 27, 1867, Lister called attention to a new method of treatment of hernias opened in the presence of atmospheric air; in September of the same year, in the same journal, we find an article by Lister "On the antiseptic principle in the practice of surgery." The spring of 1867, therefore, is the date of the beginning of the antiseptic era, since he first in this article used the word antiseptic in its present sense, a name which has been pregnant of such good influence and result.

Lister was assiduous in his efforts to perfect his method of wound-treatment based on the view of a contagium vivum, and in 1870 he presented his antiseptic dressing, which I need not describe, since it is no longer used by any surgeon, not even by Lister himself. But Lister's views in regard to the essential elements of wound treatment are still accepted, and these are:

Decomposition in a wound, and affections of wounds due to decomposition, are intimately connected with micro-organisms coming from without.

The wound treatment and dressing should prevent the access of micro-organisms, and, when these have entered notwithstanding every care, they should kill them or render them incapable of harm.

The dressing and the substance used for killing the micro-organisms should not irritate the wound at all, or, at best, very little.

The bactericide substances were called antiseptics, and there are a large number of these to-day, and new ones are daily being proposed; under such circumstances there are, of course, a large number of antiseptic dressings. Before, however, a generally useful wound-dressing was discovered, another observer was needed, who, by the acuteness of his observations and the finding of new and exact experimental methods, was able to clear the bacteriological road. This man was Robert Koch, who, by the method of pure culture, as well as by the logic of his experiments and conclusions, has solved the problem and gained adherents to his views.

An example will make the matter clear.

Koch's assumption that tuberculosis was dependent on the

tubercle bacillus was received with much doubt. After, however, he had shown that the bacillus was never lacking in a tubercular individual; further, that this micro-organism could be cultivated outside of the individual and remained ever the same, and that inoculation of an animal with a tenth or a twentieth generation would produce tuberculosis, then the doubters had to yield against their will and grant the truth of the action of the tubercle bacillus.

Koch has further determined the ability of the various antiseptic agents to kill the bacteria and to prevent their development, and thus stated their medicinal, surgical and hygienic value. He has indeed had a great influence on the furtherance of the contagium vivum doctrine, and has added nearly as much as Lister and Pasteur to the progress of antisepsis, surgery and hygiene.

The Production of Inflammation and Suppuration by Microbes.

Lister's antisepsis only proved that diseases of wounds, diphtheria of wounds, hospital gangrene, pyæmia and septicæmia were the result of fermentation and of decomposition, and that these were caused by the action of bacteria; the method of Koch proved that erysipelas and probably ordinary suppuration were dependent on bacillary infection.

Lister and his school have claimed as an antiseptic and aseptic course when a wound healed without fever, even though this was accompanied by considerable suppuration; Koch has proved that even laudable pus was due to a species of coccus.

Twenty-five years before, C. Hueter claimed that inflammation and suppuration were due to monads, and that when these were lacking then there could be neither inflammation nor suppuration; since, however, he could not clearly support this proposition, the majority of surgeons held aloof from it.

When, however, it had been proved possible to cause suppuration by the introduction of pure culture cocci; when, further, it had been proved that where stringent antiseptic precautions were taken neither mechanical, thermic nor chemical irritation and tissue wounds—as, for instance, by the introduction of sterilized glass, stone or metal—caused suppuration or inflammation, then did surgeons agree with Hueter's view, and grant that even laudable pus and its accompanying inflammation were due to cocci, and that the use of antiseptic means which killed the cocci or rendered them incapable of function would prevent these. It has, then, become an axiom that both inflammation and suppuration, as well as wound diseases, are the direct consequences of the action of micro-organisms.

This view simplifies the etiology of inflammation, suppuration and wound diseases greatly.

Now that we know that cocci, bacteria, bacilli and spirillæ are present in the earth, air and water around us; and now that from numerous observations we know that micro-organisms are absent from the fluids and tissues of healthy human and animal bodies, as well as from the fluids and tissues of sound plants, we are driven, thence, to the conclusion that the epidermis, the tissues and the fluids of animals and plants proteet against micro-organisms; and that, on the other hand, in case of wounds and surgical operations where the protecting epidermis has been injured, or when through disease the epidermis has lost its impermeability, then is the entrance of one or of many micro-organisms possible, and these cause inflammation, suppuration and the various wound diseases.

We have spoken thus far of diseases of wounds alone, but it is clear that many internal diseases may also be due to micro-organisms; and further, since we know that micro-organisms are able to cause oxidation and to increase in number, and since, too, on the surface of bare rocks and of earth and in very many internal diseases micro-organisms have been found, then we must grant that the crumbling of rocks, the withering of plants, as well as decomposition, corruption, and decay, are due to micro-organisms.

The pangermists see in micro-organisms the cause of most internal and external diseases, and claim that these are at the basis of pathology, and indeed of medical science in general; and they also lay to micro-organisms the germination of plants, and withering, decomposition, corrosion, and foulness in general. They see in the life of these workers the cause of order in growth and decay throughout organic nature.

We will not follow the pangermists in their philosophical speculations, but will pass to the consideration of our subject —the influence of micro-organisms on surgical diseases.

The Staphylococcus Pyogenes Aureus, Albus and Citreus, and the Streptococcus as the Causal Factors of Suppuration and of Wound Diseases.

Towards the diagnosis of the different kinds of pathogenetic microbes and their relation to various surgical diseases much is as yet lacking, and there is considerable difference of opinion.

From the observations of Ogston, Rosenbach, Carré and others, it is known that every kind of pus contains a micro-organism, which Ogston, owing to its racemose shape, has called the staphylococcus. This coccus has the peculiarity, when cultivated on gelatin plates, of developing a beautiful orange-yellow pigment, and when man is inoculated with it it causes suppuration. He gave the name of staphylococcus pyogenes aureus to this coccus on account of the above peculiarity. This coccus is widely disseminated through the atmosphere and singularly resistant to reagents; it may be dried, baked, treated to chemical reagents, and yet be neither killed nor deprived of its properties. It is hence conceivable why, after wounds, inflammation and suppuration so frequently set in, and why the staphylococcus pyogenes aureus is found as the causal factor of the pus. This micro-organism, however, is not the only one found in pus. Rosenbach has discovered, as well, a staphylococcus pyogenes albus and Passet a staphylococcus pyogenes citreus.

As to whether these three cocci, which are differentiated the one from the other only by the fact that they develop pigments, are the same or different species we cannot with certainty state; the white and the citron-yellow are, however, much less frequently found than the golden. Even the golden works in different ways: It only causes pus when inoculated in man; animals cannot be inoculated. In animals the staphylococcus pyogenes aureus must be placed under the skin or in a serous cavity in order to cause pus. In case it is directly injected into the blood, it causes the characteristic, dangerous form of endocarditis ulcerosa; when, however, the staphylococcus aureus is injected into the blood of an animal which has broken or injured its leg then it causes an osteomyelitis. If this micro-parasite, furthermore, is injected into the lymph channels, then it causes metastatic abscesses in the liver, kidneys, etc., as also suppuration in the joints. Likely enough these metastases in various organs and in the joints, the osteomyelitis and the ulcerative endocarditis, would be caused in man by the staphylococcus pyogenes aureus even as they are in animals upon which we experiment.

In addition to the staphylococcus pyogenes there is another micro-parasite which causes suppuration, although it is rarely met with. It is a coccus made up of small rings linked together in a chain. It is called streptococcus pyogenes, and is readily differentiated from the staphylococcus pyogenes. This coccus, or one so like it that differentiation is not possible, has been found by Fehleisen in the borders of an erysipelatous patch. Fehleisen has cultivated this coccus, and was able with any generation to cause a typical erysipelas.

THE QUESTION OF ANTISEPSIS.

It is quite evident that there exist a number of micro-parasites which are in a position to cause inflammation and suppuration. We witness daily the fact that one and the same effect may be the outcome of different causes. It is less evident why the same coccus should now cause simple suppuration, and next pus metastases or osteomyelitis, or ulcerative endocarditis, or again typical erysipelas.

Since now we have shown that inflammation, suppuration and different wound diseases are caused by micro-organisms, it follows as a consequence that the therapeutic aim must be to kill these microbes. This essential, however, is a difficult one to satisfy. When the microbes have once entered the body and have there taken their abode, then we have no certain means of dislodging or of killing them without at the same time injuring this body. In the body we can only prevent or limit their development and weaken their injurious action; it is, however, always possible for the weakened coccus to unexpectedly recover its vitality.

Our treatment then must aim at not allowing the microbes to enter the body. Since, however, the microbes exist everywhere—in the air, on our hands, clothing, instruments, bandages, etc., therefore is it necessary to operate, to dress, and to change the dressings of the wounds under careful antiseptic precautions.

ANTISEPTIC OPERATIONS.

To-day antisepsis is practiced as follows: The operating room has smooth, polished walls and a so-called asphalt floor. The walls and floor can and must be washed and cleansed before each operation. The surgeon, his assistants and the nurses must wash and brush their hands with soap and water and disinfect them in a 2 per cent. carbolic solution or in a $\frac{1}{2}$ per cent. sublimate solution; their usual clothes should be removed, and clean operating coats should be put on. The instruments required for operation should be jointless (with nickel-plated or hard rubber handles) and should be soaked for half an hour before the operation in a porcelain basin filled with a 5 per cent. carbolic solution. The patient should be washed at the operation-site with soap and brush and then disinfected with sublimate or carbolic. If the site is hairy it should be shaved. When the operation-site is covered with dried pus or scabs these should be loosened with turpentine or benzine and removed. To remove blood small wads of sterilized cotton or gauze, or sponges which have been soaked in 5 per cent. carbolic, should be used.

As yet Schede's method of leaving alone whatever small vessels are cut during the operation and of not washing away the blood which has oozed has not gained acceptance. On the contrary, it is customary to ligate or to twist every bleeding vessel, and to wash away the blood which otherwise it is feared would degenerate. Still, since the blood left in the wound is far less likely to decompose than the blood serum, the issue of which from the tissues cannot be prevented, some surgeons, notably J. Wolf of Berlin and myself, are in the habit of only ligating the larger vessels which happen to be cut. I use in my operations the peroxide of hydrogen, with the double aim of causing contraction of the lumen of the cut vessels and of preventing decomposition of the blood and serum. Schede's method, however, although not generally accepted, has had a good influence over the too careful ligating methods of certain surgical schools.

After the completion of the operation the wound should be washed for from one to two minutes with a 2 to 3 per cent. carbolic solution. This latter manipulation aims at killing or rendering inert any microbes in the wound.

The above directions are followed by all surgeons who operate antiseptically.

SYNOPSIS OF THE CHIEF ANTISEPTICS USED BEFORE AND SINCE THE ANTISEPTIC ERA, AND THEIR VALUE.

I desire, before pursuing this study further, to consider here the chief and most useful antiseptics, from the earliest times to date, in connection with their chemical composition, structure (as far as I am familiar with this), their peculiarities and their dosage.

I will consider as obsolete the great majority of antiseptic dressings, the antiseptic plasters and salves and balsams of the older surgeons, and refer only to the following:

1. *Aqua picis,* or tar water, which is prepared by dissolving one part of tar in five to six parts of water. In twelve to fifteen hours the solution is complete, as far as this is possible. 2. The *aqua vulneraria spirituosa* was obtained by the distillation of alcoholic fluid from different plants. 3. The wine and camphor-containing dressings. 4. The juice of oleaginous, aromatic and tonic plants. 5. The *aquæ plumbica, saturnina, vegeto-mineris, Goulardi,* etc.

In 1854 Burrow proposed as an active antiseptic what is known in the German pharmacopeia as the liquor alumini acetici. The formula is $Al_2 (CH_0 COO)_4 (OH)_2$. This combination is a difficult one and not stable. Latterly Athenstädt has proposed the following formula, which is readily soluble in water, and not poisonous:

Alumin-acetico-tartarici,	.	gr. xxx.–xlv.
Aquæ distillat.,	. . . .	℥ iij. ℨ j.

In 1806 Freiherrn v. Reichenbach recommended creasote for dressings. This is a complicated body, the chemical combination of which is not exactly known to me, although I have used it for a number of years.

A few years later carbolic acid was proposed, and Lister has greatly popularized its use.

Pure carbolic acid is not an aromatic acid but rather an alcohol. Its chemical name is phenol, or phenyl-alcohol, and its formula is $C_6H_5 (OH)$. The uses of carbolic are so well known that it is unnecessary to dwell on them here.

15

The use of phenol led to that of many other antiseptics which are more powerful in less concentration. We will only briefly refer to the following:

Salicylic acid, the chemical formula of which is C_6H_4 (HO) (COOH), is soluble in 300 parts of water and is a very powerful antiseptic.

Next comes sozol-acid, also called aseptol. Its formula is:

$$C_6H_4 \begin{cases} OH \\ SO_3H. \end{cases}$$

It is prepared by mixing equal parts of phenol and concentrated sulphuric acid. After two to three days' rest and neutralization by the carbonate of barium, a $33\frac{1}{3}$ per cent. solution of aseptol is obtained, which is soluble in any proportion in water and is neither poisonous nor irritating to the body even when concentrated. I have used aseptol in 5 per cent. solution, but cannot say that it possesses any advantages over phenol or salicylic acid; its sole advantage, possibly, is its usefulness as an antiseptic in eye diseases, where both carbolic and salicylic acids are not readily applicable.

Analogous in its action to aseptol is resorcin (metadioxy-benzol) proposed by Hlassiwetz and Barth.

$$C_6H_4 \begin{cases} OH\ 1 \\ OH\ 3. \end{cases}$$

A 1 to 2 per cent. solution is not poisonous as an eye-wash, for inhalations and dressings.

Hydrochinon (paradioxybenzol) has the formula

$$C_6H_4 \begin{cases} OH\ 1 \\ OH\ 4, \end{cases}$$

and has not been used as a surgical antiseptic notwithstanding its anti-fermentative properties.

If equal parts of pure anilin ($C_6H_5NH_2$) and glacial acetic acid be boiled for two days we obtain a fatty-feeling body in the shape of colorless crystalline plates. This is acetanilid,

$$(C_6H_4NH\ (CH_0\ CO),$$

which Kussmaul has given in typhus, intermittent, pneumonia in four grain doses as an antipyretic—whence its name anti-febrin.

This is soluble in about 200 parts water, and I have used it in this concentration as well as in powder form as an antiseptic.

I was unable to determine any advantage it possessed over the previously mentioned antiseptics.

On the other hand I have found antipyrin, proposed by Ludwig Knorr in 1884, superior. All antiseptics, in addition to their bactericide properties, possess the power of preventing decomposition and fermentation and of quieting pain, as well as in a measure lowering fever. Antipyrin, while equal to other antiseptics in its property of preventing decomposition and fermentation, as a local anodyne is not approached by any others, and as an external antipyretic it is as powerful as salicylic acid.

The chemical name of antipyrin is dimethyloxylchinicin, and its formula $C_{11}H_{12}N_2O$.

Antipyrin is soluble in equal parts of water, alcohol, or chloroform, and with difficulty in ether. It is most valuable as a local anodyne, as an antiseptic, as a local antipyretic, as also for incorporation in dressings. Its high cost, however, prevents its routine use.

Skraup has synthetically constructed out of anilin, nitro-benzol, glycerin, and sulphuric acid what he has termed chinolin (C_9H_7N). This body is readily soluble in alcohol, ether, chloroform and benzine, but with difficulty in water; according to Donat it is a very useful antiseptic in watery solution. In a 2 per cent. solution it controls decomposition of urine and of fæces; in 4 per cent. solution it prevents blood decomposition; in 1 per cent. solution it prevents the coagulation of blood and of albumin.

It has been used as a local applicant in diphtheria, and as a mouth and tooth wash in the following solutions:

℞ Chinolini pur., ... gr. xxxvij.
  Spts, vini gall.,
  Aq. distillat., . . . āā ℥ j. ℨ vj.
  S. For local use.

℞ Chinolini, ... gr. x.-xv.
  Spts. vini gall., ... ℥ j. ℨ vj.
  Aq. distillat., ... Oj.
  Ol. menth. pip., ... gtt. 2 to 3.
  S. To be used as a gargle.

The following salts of chinolin, owing to their greater solubility in water, are useful in surgery: chinolin-salicylat, chino-

lin-salicylic acid (C_9H_7N, $C_7H_6O_3$), chinolin-tartrate, and the
vinegar of chinolin, 3 (C_9H_7N), 4 ($C_4H_6O_6$).

I have only used, as an injection in gonorrhœa, the following formula:

> ℞ Chinolin tartarici, ... **gr. xv.**
> Aq. distillat., ... ℥ iv. ℨ vj.
> S. To be used as an injection.

and I have found it more effective than the usual zinc, silver
and permanganate of potass solutions.

Finally, we must refer to sublimate, the best of all antiseptics.

I would here notice the complaint that sublimate, which in
solution of 1 to 50,000 is still antiseptic, sometimes fails the
surgeon when in solution of 1 to 1000. It appears that 7 minims
of bullock serum added to 7 minims of 1 to 1000 sublimate
solution, takes away the antiseptic property, the sublimate
being rendered insoluble by the serum. To avoid this Dr. E.
Laplace, of New Orleans, has suggested the acidification of the
sublimate solution.

To prepare an antiseptic sublimate solution Laplace orders:

> Hydrarg. bi-chlor.,.   .   .   .   . **gr. xv.**
> Acid. tartaric., ... ℨ j. gr. xv.
> Aq. distillat., ... Oij.

To prepare an antiseptic gauze solution he orders:

> Hydrarg. bi-chlor., ... ℨ j. gr. xv.
> Acid. tartaric., ... ℨ v.
> Aquæ distillat., ... Oij.

These formulæ are being now used in Bergmann's clinic,
and they seem to be the best of all for surgical use. Personally I do not use these formulæ, for the reason that I no longer
resort to sublimate but to other antiseptics.

I desire still to briefly refer to antiseptic dressings containing powdered drugs.

I have covered wounds with the powder of a large number
of plants and chemical substances, placing a gauze bandage
over all. I have thus used the pulv. irid. florentin., the pulv.
rad. altheæ, and liquiritiæ, the finely powdered kolophonium

and sanguis draconis, the powdered zinc oxide and pure salicylic acid.

These dry powders gave me much satisfaction; the objection to the salicylic acid was the fact that for five minutes after its application it caused intense burning, and in sensitive patients this lasted even for an hour and longer. To avoid this I have mixed the salicylic powder with 3 to 5 per cent. of an indifferent powder. Thus:

Acid. salicylic.	. . . . .	gr. xv.
Ox. zinci .	. . . . . .	gr. xlv.
Talci venet.,	. . . . . .	℥ vj. gr. xvj.

is a combination which has yielded excellent results in case of atonic ulcers, especially those of the lower extremities.

I have also used soluble powders over wounds. Thus, chloral hydrate, different metallic salts with 1 to 3 per cent. of indifferent powders (chalk, magnesium, etc.), have been tested. I have found that all antiseptics can thus be used in powder form; even sublimate may be mixed with chalk in the proportion of 1:1000.

This method of mine of using antiseptics in powder led to the suggestion of many combinations, of which I will mention a few.

Mosetig v. Moorhof has used iodoform as a wound dressing on the strength of the strong recommendation of Moleschott, who gave it internally. He spreads the iodoform powder over the wound even as I had done with the salicylic acid powder. He has found that it checks hemorrhage and pain, controls suppuration and cures local tuberculosis. He later impregnated gauze with a 10 to 50 per cent. solution of iodoform in alcohol and ether. Finally he mixed iodoform with equal parts of collodion to form an iodoform-collodion for the skin around wounds.

Iodoform quickly secured the approbation of surgeons the world over. It has, however, great disadvantages. Thus: The penetrating smell of iodoform cannot be disguised, and this smell is to many unbearable. Some individuals are poisoned by the agent; they lose their appetite, become morose, absent-minded, and if the action be continued there result psychical troubles and death. Skilful observers have claimed that the agent is neither antiseptic nor bactericide.

v. Mosetig has modified his early practice. He now only spreads a small quantity of iodoform on the wound and covers this over with iodoform gauze. The objections to the agent still hold, however. I would recommend the following formula:

Iodoform, ... gr. xv.–xlv.
Talc. venen., ... ℥ iij. ℈ j.

Many substitutes for iodoform have latterly been proposed. In the first rank we note tetraiodpyrrol or iodol, as it has been called.

In 1885 iodol was prepared by Ciamician and Silber by the mixture of pyrrol (C_4H_5N) with an alcoholic solution of iodine. It is a yellow, odorless and tasteless, crystalline powder, almost insoluble in water (1 in 5000), in ether in equal parts, in alcohol in three parts, in oil in fifteen. It is not poisonous.

It may be used as a powder:

Iodol, ... ℈ j. gr. xv.
Talc. venet., ... ℥ iij. ℈ j.

As a solution:

Iodol, ... ℈ ss.
Spts. vini dil., ... ℥ j.
Glycerin, ... ℥ j. ℈ vj.
Aq. distill. . . . . . . ℥ iij. ℈ j.

As a gauze:

Iodol,
Colofonii, ... āā gr. xlv.
Glycerin., ... ℥ j. ℈ vj.
Spts. vini dil., ... ℈ iiss.
Aq. distill., ... ℥ iij. ℈ j.

the gauze being impregnated with this.

As a collodion:

Iodol, ... ℈ iiss.
Spts. vini rectif., ... ℥ iv. ℈ vj.
Pyroxylini, ... ℥ j. ℈ vj.
Ol. ricini, ... ℥ j. ℈ vj.
Aether sulph., ... ℥ ij. gr. xv.

In 1887 O. Lassar, Berlin, called attention to sozoiodol, proposed by Tromsdorff, of Erfurt, as a substitute for iodoform. Its empirical formula is $C_6H_3ISO_3$ (OH), and in chemical structure it is paraiodphenolsulphonic acid:

$$C_6H_3 \begin{cases} OH \\ \quad SO_3H \\ I \end{cases}$$

It is a beautiful yellow, odorless powder, soluble in water and alcohol, not decomposed by light, crystalline, and not poisonous. It may be used in 5 per cent. solution, or in 5 per cent. mixture with chalk.

At present the price of iodol and of sozoiodol is higher than iodoform, which has latterly fallen very low.

Kocher has had less good results with his bismuth powder than Mosetig with iodoform. Still, in the clinic at Bern the results have been as favorable; elsewhere, however, bismuth is rarely used.

Lister has suggested the oxi-iodide, or sub-iodide of bismuth. This is a heavy, crystalline, reddish-yellow, odorless powder, not soluble in water, which Lister says is an excellent antiseptic against pus, and he prefers it to iodoform. It is not poisonous.

Since it is not soluble in water, it seems to me that the gauze is not to be recommended. The bismuth-salicylate, on the contrary, is stable when treated to alcohol and ether, the acid not being driven off as is the iodine in the former gauze. It contains one-quarter of its weight of salicylic acid and three-quarters of oxide of bismuth. It may be powdered over wounds even as iodoform.

A further substitute for iodoform is phenylsalicylate, proposed by Nencky. It is known as salol in medicine and has the formula:

$$C_6H_4 \begin{cases} OH \\ COOC_6H_5 \end{cases}$$

It is a white, transparent, insoluble in water, slightly aromatic, tasteless, crystalline powder, which may be used over wounds in a 5 to 10 per cent. mixture. It is also used as a mouth wash.

℞ Saloli, ... ℨ j.– ℨ iiss.
   Talc., ... ℥ iij.– ℥ iij. ℨ ij.
   S. Externally.

℞ Saloli, ... gr. xlv.
  Spts. vin. dil., ... ℥ iij. ʒ j.
  Ol. menth. pip.,
  Ol. rosarum, ... āā gtt. 3
  S. Mouth wash, ten to fifteen drops in a glass of water.

As before remarked, any soluble or insoluble antiseptic, if only mixed in 1 to 5 per cent. proportion with an indifferent insoluble agent, may be readily used as a powder over wounds. Such being the case the number of antiseptic powders has rapidly increased. Antifebrin, antipyrin, chinolin and its salts, kairin, thallin and its salts, and many other benzol derivatives, have been made into wound powders.

Finally, I would mention as an antiseptic the fluoro-silicate of soda. Its formula is Na_2SiF_6. I do not know who first called attention to the antiseptic properties of this inorganic body. I have obtained it from Engel, in Vienna, and have tested its bactericide properties. I prepared 2 to 5 per cent. mixtures of gelatin with the agent, sterilized it and then inoculated it with full-grown yeast spores. I began with the 5 per cent., and this remained free from germs; the same happened with the 2 per cent. These data establish it as one of the few inorganic chemical antiseptics. Owing to its difficult solubility it can only be used in 1 to 1.5 per cent. solution. It should be stated that in the text-books it is said to be readily soluble, but the specimen I obtained was only so to the extent of .8 per cent. Further researches may prove it to be of great value, especially in pediatrics and in gynecology, where, owing to its odorless and non-poisonous nature and to its cheapness, it might take the place of carbolic.

It may be used in solution:

Sod. fluor. silici, ... gr. xv.–xxij.
Aquæ distillat., ... ℥ iij. ʒ j.
S. Mouth wash.

Or in powder:
Sod. fluor.-silici, ... ʒ j. gr. xv.
Talc. ven., ... ℥ iij. ʒ j.

In an operation for adeno-sarcoma of the breast and in case of many ulcers the above powder was very satisfactory. I strongly recommend it to the experience of others.

Possibly, silicium tri-iodide (Si_2I_6) recommended by Friedel, and silicico-iodoform ($SiHI_3$), might be of surgical utility.

It is apparent from the context what a large number of antiseptics are at the disposal of the surgeon. It is certainly easier to discover a new antiseptic than to find the requisite number of wounds on which to test the new antiseptics. It would take more than ten years to weigh the value of those we already have. In these pages I could only refer to those best known and most useful to the practical surgeon.

ANTISEPTIC DRESSING, DRAINAGE, SUTURE, PERMANENT DRESSING AND KREOLIN.

All modern surgeons have the same aims in their dressings. The wound should, if possible, not suppurate, and there should be no secretion, but if suppuration cannot be prevented then decomposition and fermentation should be guarded against. The dressing, further, during union, should protect the wound against the entrance of microbes and also against various other harmful influences. ·

These aims may be reached in a number of ways.

A small number of surgeons use the simple iodoform gauze dressing. The surroundings of the wound are painted with iodoform collodion (1 to 10 or 15). In the wound a rolled piece of iodoform gauze is laid; the wound is then covered with ten to twenty folds of the gauze, over this a layer of absorbent cotton about 2 inches thick, and then a strip of muslin is rolled over all. A few surgeons use pure iodoform powder or a mixture with zinc-oxide, magnesia, chalk, etc.; others use pure salicylic acid or a mixture of this with zinc-oxide, etc.; others salol, and other bactericide substances. Over the powder they lay gauze, absorbent cotton, and fix all in place with gauze or an ordinary roller bandage.

The majority of practicing physicians use the sublimate dressing in the same way as formerly the carbolic and salicylic dressings were used. To carry off the secretion from the wound for one to six days, one or more drainage tubes are placed in the wound. Over the wound a thick layer ($\frac{1}{2}$ inch) of a 1 per cent. sublimate gauze is laid; over this a layer of absorbent cotton; over this a piece of mackintosh or gutta-percha paper; and all is held in place by a roller bandage.

Before I proceed to a description of the various antiseptics I must say a few words about drainage.

It is well known to the older surgeons that in pre-antiseptic times the number of cases of suppuration and of pyæmia was considerably lessened by the introduction of drainage, and that even the advent of the antiseptic era could not entirely banish drainage. I consider, therefore, the drainage tube an excellent antiseptic adjuvant.

Many attempts have been made to substitute something else for the rubber drainage tubes introduced by Chassaignac. Hueter has recommended silver and glass drains; Lister, horse hair; Watson-Cheyne, catgut; I have used goldbeaters' skins rolled together like a tube, and asbestos lint; Gersuny, iodoform threadlets; Billroth, iodoform-tannin pencils. All these, however, have not been able to displace rubber drain tubes.

Since drain tubes are used as antiseptics, it may be thought that these should, or must, remain in place till union is complete. Not so; in the majority of cases they have played their part in one to six days, and they may then be removed.

The fact cannot too often be emphasized that of all animal albumin-containing fluids the serum from the surface of wounds most readily decomposes, and that only the first stage of this process bodes ill to the health and the life of the wounded subject; and further that the drain tube answers the purpose of carrying away from the wound the serum which collects after any injury. Drainage tubes are, therefore, only requisite in the period which precedes suppuration—that is to say, during the first six days after the injury.

While in use the drain tube converts the occlusion method of treating wounds into a partially open method. When the period of suppuration has become established, then the drain tube is not only not necessary, but it becomes a foreign body and prevents union. The drain tube left *in situ* too long is even as harmful as the too strong application of carbolic acid, and should, therefore, be forbidden. Only exceptionally is it desirable to leave the drain tube in during suppuration; when, for instance, there is sacculation of the pus, then will the tube answer the purpose of preventing this. Retention of pus, however, is an abnormal process in a wound, for when matters are progressing favorably this should not occur. Formation of pus and depuration in normal cases balance one another; only abnormal irritation increases the wound secretion and this may lead to retention of pus.

Retention of pus, then, in normal cases must be considered an exception. These exceptions, however, cannot formulate any rule for normal cases, and in the latter, then, the tube should be removed in from one to six days.

The use of the drainage tube is unnecessary in the following cases:

In the open wound treatment.

In case of flat wounds, where the dressing can soak up the secretion and carry it off.

In cavity wounds, which can be thoroughly tamponed and thus are converted practically into flat wounds.

In cases where the intention is to bring the edges together only after the lapse of one to three days.

Ten to fifteen years ago, when I used the écraseur and the cautery a great deal, I came to the conclusion that in order to obtain union by first intention sharply defined wound-margins were not essential; for the margins cut by the écraseur or by the cautery knife healed as readily. I have also brought suppurating wounds together by suture, without first freshening the edges, and I have often thus obtained union in suppurating wounds of the face. I have also obtained union by the insertion of sutures twenty-four to forty-eight hours after the operation.

The late suture, that inserted during the stage of suppuration, is called the secondary suture. In the use of this, drainage may ordinarily be dispensed with. We must note the fact, however, that the secondary suture, which occasionally is to be preferred to the primary, is contra-indicated in laparotomy for reasons which need not detain us here.

After this digression I proceed to a consideration of the concentration and the preparation of sublimate. This is prepared with alcohol and glycerin, with salt and glycerin in varying strengths of 1 to 300 to 2000.

v. Bergmann, the first and the warmest advocate of sublimate, uses a solution of 10 parts sublimate, 500 glycerin, 1000 alcohol and 1500 distilled water, over about 70 yards of gauze; this gauze when freshly dried contains about $\frac{1}{3}$ per cent. sublimate. Maase takes $\mathfrak{z}$ j. $\mathfrak{z}$ v.j. of sublimate, 1 quart of boiled water, $6\frac{2}{3}$ pounds of salt dissolved in 10 quarts of water; these are mixed, filtered, and to the filtrate 1200 parts of glycerin are added. This solution will impregnate 270 yards of gauze. Lister uses 2.5 parts of sublimate and 1 part of salmiac to 5000 of water. When Koch determined that sublimate was effective in the strength of 1 to 20,000, and that solutions of 1 to 300,000 prevented the development of microbes, then it became apparent that solutions of 1 to 2000 to 5000 could be used for impregnating gauze. Some surgeons use a combination of all possible antiseptics. Iodoform, carbolic, salicylic, and sublimate gauzes are used together; others still use protecting silk, cotton, etc. Such a cumulation and combination is not at all necessary, and very expensive.

I must still refer to an antiseptic which is superior to others. The number at our disposal is indeed too great. v. Mussbaum collected 80 agents, and of these only a few were generally known. As early as 1865 I used creasote, and specially referred to it in my work on military surgery, which appeared in 1866. I used this agent exclusively up to 1873, for I found that it acted better than carbolic. In 1875 I gave it up because other surgeons deemed it inferior to carbolic. P. Guttman has latterly tested its antiseptic properties after Koch's method, and I am pleased to find that he ranks it higher than carbolic. Carbolic acid is likely to evoke toxic symptoms; it injures the hands of the surgeon and takes the edge off his instruments. For awhile it was replaced by salicylic acid, and then these by iodoform; the latter, on account of its odor and its tendency to affect the intellect, was replaced by the long-known sublimate.

We possess now another antiseptic which may displace all hitherto used antiseptics, even carbolic and salicylic acids, iodoform and sublimate, and this is kreolin, a preparation obtained by dry distillation from English coal, which has the following characteristics: It is absolutely non-toxic in man and the higher animals, but for the microbes it is ten times more deadly than carbolic acid; it is soluble in water, alcohol and glycerin; it controls hemorrhage and pain; it limits suppuration; it injures neither metals nor the hands, but cleanses, disinfects and preserves both; it is very cheap. So far no disadvantages have been determined. We trust therefore that it will soon be accepted in surgery.[1] As to how long it will hold this position in this age of progress it is not possible to say.

---

[1] See the "Internationale Klinische Rundschau," Nos. 1 and 3, 1888.

In these pages we have always spoken of gauze for the dressing because it is the most convenient. There are many other agents, however, which are used as dressings. As to whether one or another is resorted to will depend on the choice of the individual, the question of cost, etc. All the materials in routine use are readily sterilized and impregnated with antiseptic fluids.

A few words now in regard to the change of dressings.

In the days when it was the belief that salves, plasters and topical applications had an active influence in causing union, it was deemed requisite to change the dressing frequently, and since then pus was considered to interfere with healing, the aim was to wash this away by permanent irrigation or warm baths. The bad results obtained from the latter means led surgeons to a simple change in the dressings, in private practice three to four times daily, and in hospitals once to twice. To change the dressing less than once was considered bad practice. When in 1859 I was called upon to attend so many serious wounds that it was physically impossible to change all the dressings daily, I divided the wounded in two groups, and in one or the other did not change the dressings for one or more days. When I found that the wounds which were left alone had a better appearance than those which were changed daily it became my custom to re-dress all wounds less frequently, that is every second to fourth day.

After I had used creasote for six years I was able to obtain union of large wounds by only dressing three to four times. I have since followed this practice, having learned that frequent change was injurious and unnecessary. I even went so far as to leave the dressing untouched for ten to fourteen days and then found the wound nearly or entirely healed.

A few years ago Neuber gave to this method the name of the permanent dressing. The child having been named, surgeons have considered the method a legitimate one in the treatment of wounds. It remains, then, only for me to state the limits of time during which the dressing may remain. For the present neither the days nor the weeks can be definitely stated. A permanent dressing may be defined as one which is only renewed when necessary, in opposition to the previous method where the change was made without stringent call, or because it was the custom to do so daily in order to observe the progress of healing. From my stand-point, rather than speak of a permanent dressing, I prefer the term obligatory change of dressing, as being more defining than the term permanent. The necessity or the advisability of a change of dressing depends on the following circumstances:

1. When the patient complains of pain in the wound or dragging, then, whether the dressing has been in place a few days or a few hours, it should be changed.

2. When the patient is feverish, loses flesh and strength without evident cause, then the dressing must be changed, since the source of the disturbance may be in the wound.

3. When neither pain nor fever but profuse suppuration is present; when, in consequence, the wound stinks and thus inconveniences and disturbs the patient, then must the dressing be altered, no matter how long it has been *in situ.* When the dressing is only soiled by pus without otherwise interfering with the patient, then it is customary to change the dressing for æsthetic reasons—although I do not grant the urgency here, for all a man has to do is to throw a roller gauze bandage over the soiled dressing without disturbing the wound and yet complying with the demands of æstheticism.

We desire to emphasize the fact that a change in the dressing before complete healing of the wound, however carefully this is attended to, carries with it still a greater or less irritation, and therefore this should, when possible, be avoided. The obligatory dressing outweighs any objection, and is stringently called for. In any individual case the limitations of a single dressing will be apparent.

Every form of dressing, and there are more than 100, gives equally good results. The majority of wounds heal under all these dressings by first intention. Aggravated wound disease is to-day rarely seen, and it must be granted that the doctrine of a contagium animatum has had a healthy and a beneficial effect on surgery and on humanity.

THE EXISTENCE OF PHAGOCYTES, OF PTOMAINES AND OF LEUCOMAINES ARE ESSENTIAL HYPOTHESES FOR THE EXPLANATION OF MANY PHENOMENA.

The good results obtained in the healing of wounds should not blind us in the search for the true explanation of the factor, and not cause us to abstain from the determination of the truth. The fact that the so-called open treatment of wounds, where all sorts of micro-organisms have free access, gives as good results as the antiseptic occlusion method, evokes the query as to whether the conclusions drawn from the theory of a contagium vivum will apply to all the phenomena, and as to whether the observations may not receive their sufficient explanation from the stand-point of some other theory? There are a large number of phenomena which are not completely explained by the antiseptic theory. A few examples will suffice:

All surgeons are in accord in regard to the worth of iodoform in checking pus formation and in assisting granulation, while all observers agree that iodoform neither kills nor controls the powers of bacteria.

The inoculation of pathogenetic bacteria is followed by no results in many animals and in many men, while decomposed fluids which have been deprived of microbes by filtration or boiling retain their poisonous properties on the bodies of animals.

These and other facts render resort to other hypotheses necessary. One of these is that of Metschikoff, who, from microscopical examinations, evolved the hypothesis of phagocytes, which makes the object and aim of the white blood corpuscles to swallow and kill the bacteria. When the latter invade the body in very large numbers, when the bacteria in number and strength are more powerful, then the white blood corpuscles are killed by the bacteria.

Another hypothesis is the following: We have often referred to the fact that fermentation, necrosis and decomposition are the result of the action of micro-organisms. When microbes are lacking or interfered with in development, then neither fermentation nor decomposition occurs. It is supposed, then, that these microbes, which are nourished at the expense of the albumin of the body, are dissolved by it. In the process of this solution materials are formed, called ptomaïnes, which have the property, even as have alkaloids or poisons in relatively slight amount, to poison and to have a deadly effect on animal bodies.

Gautier has shown that in the discharges of entirely healthy animals, poisonous, alkaloid-like bodies are to be found which are not products of decomposition, and which he has called

leucomaines. He has found this alkaloid in the saliva, urine,
etc., of animals. From the muscle of larger animals he has obtained five different crystalline alkaloids (leucomaines), which
were very acid and acted as poisons on the nerve centres.
These leucomaines belong to the ptomaïne group, and they are
both found in animal bodies. Their number is now more than
thirty.

According to these hypotheses it is not absolutely essential that decomposition bacteria should be brought to the body
which is infected; it is sufficient if their products of decomposition are brought. The bacteria themselves may be killed or
removed by filtration.

The existence of these ptomaïnes is testified to by such men
as Panum, Selmi, Brieger, Nencki, Bergmann, Schmiedeberg,
Zuelzer, Sonnenschein, Guareschi, Mosso, Gautier, and others.

THE PRESENT VIEW OF THE ACTION OF MICROBES.

From the foregoing, the present opinion in regard to the influence of microbes on the development of inflammation, of
suppuration and of wound diseases may be gathered. This
view, in its present form, was not reached of a sudden, but has
slowly developed, and it will not probably remain as at present
established. A long time elapsed from Hueter's personally
expressed opinion that neither inflammation nor suppuration
could occur without the action of monads to the finding of the
staphylo- and strepto-coccus pyogenes and their acceptance
by surgeons. We must still point out how the theory of a
contagium animatum began to spread, and what influence the
change of opinion had on our present view.

It is and remains a fact that micro-organisms can cause
wound diseases; the query now is how they do this? It is
claimed that this occurs through their unlimited increase in
a mechanical way, through stoppage of capillaries, or through
solution of albumin, or in a chemical way.

According to the teachings and the axioms of physiology,
however, mechanical and chemical agents do not act directly
on the body. All processes in man, as in animals, in health
as well as in disease, progress only under the influence of
nerves. It is the sympathetic nerves, the vaso-motors, which
actively contract and dilate the capillaries, and thus render the
lumina narrower or wider, and assist the diffusion of fluids or

gases, preventing or increasing this. It is the vaso-constrictors and the vaso-dilators which preside over interchange in the body, equilibrating the nutrition, or interfering with it, and thus leading to disease.

Local mechanical and chemical agents work only indirectly through the sympathetic nerves on the body; and the microbes can only indirectly work ill by irritating the sympathetic nerves into a diseased state. The entrance of bacteria into the body and their residence there and means of support, effect an irritation which the sympathetic nerves receive, and this leads to afflux of blood to the irritated part owing to the dilatation of innervated capillaries. The congestion, the stasis, the altered local diffusion and nutrient phenomena, are the natural consequences of the local irritation, and when this local irritation with its consequences is of long standing, then general disturbances of nutrition occur in the body—that is to say, diseases.

At once we see that this view of the cause of wound diseases is very similar to that of physicians of olden time. The early physicians claimed that inflammation, suppuration and wound diseases were due to an irritation of the sympathetic and trophic nerves, and that this led to a disturbance of the healthy equilibrium. To them the irritant was a mechanical, thermic or chemical one; to us the entrance and action of microbes in the body and the resulting nutrition changes are the cause.

The difference between these two views is that whereas the older physicians claimed that mechanical, thermic and chemical irritants caused disease, the modern physicians admit only microbes; they grant the effect of mechanical, thermic and chemical causes only in so far as these assist the entrance of microbes into the body; when the latter are prevented from entering the body, then neither mechanical, chemical nor thermic effects alone are able of themselves to cause inflammation, suppuration and wound diseases.

Consequences Resulting from the Prevailing Theory.

It might seem as if the prevailing theory, which states that the microbes are only to be regarded as irritants of the sympathetic and trophic nerves, does not assist our pathological knowledge or the truth, seeing that the manner in which the sympathetic and trophic nerves alter the calibre of the blood-vessels, and thus assist or limit the diffusion of gases and of fluids, is as little known and explainable as the theory of the direct action of microbes on the tissue.   But this is not so.

It is certainly progress in our knowledge of pathological processes when we recognize that the same factors which regulate the calibre of the capillaries and the nutrient changes in the healthy body act in the same way in the abnormal state of disease.

As to the manner in which the sympathetic nerves alter the calibre of the capillaries and the nutrient changes in the tissues, we do know something about this, and it is explainable.   It is as clear and comprehensible as the process by which the dynamo in its 500 revolutions to the minute yields light, heat, chemical and mechanical work.

In both instances, by the working of the sympathetic nerves on the capillaries and on the nutrient changes, even as by the rotation of the dynamo light, warmth and chemical action result, we are dealing with what physicists call transformation of energy.

The view that the micro-organisms do not cause wound diseases directly, but only through the medium of the sympathetic nerves, is a still further advance in our knowledge.

Every layman knows that shame, anger, terror and disease may cause redness or pallor of the face, that the sight of certain foods and drinks, indeed even the mere thought sometimes, will excite the salivary glands to greater secretion and cause the mouth to be filled to overflowing.   We know that anger causes the venom-glands of the snake to fill, and that from simple sight, smell or handling the corpora cavernosa penis becomes congested with blood and sometimes even the semen is ejaculated.   That such effects are not due to the action of germs even the most rabid pangermist will grant; they are to be considered as due to the sympathetic nerves, which are irritated, and thence reflexively ensue changes in the lumina of the capillaries and nutrient changes.

Since we know, however, that sympathetic nerves may be irritated by various agents, and that as a result of any irritation hyperæmia, stasis and disturbances of nutrition may result, we cannot say that micro-organisms alone may give rise to such effects; we must thus express ourselves: Inflammation and suppuration may be caused by the staphylo- and the strepto-coccus, but also by other irritants of the sympathetic nerves.

In medicine the error is not infrequently made of considering the great majority of logical categories as absolute, while in reality only a small number of them are. When, for example, it is claimed that a foreign body in the trachea will cause dyspnœa and suffocation, it must not thence be inferred that when dyspnœa and suffocation are present there is present a foreign body in the trachea. A tetanus or a paralysis of the essential respiratory muscles may give rise to dyspnœa and to suffocation, and yet the lumen of the trachea is not obstructed in any way. A paralysis or a paresis of the heart, whereby the blood cannot be driven through the lungs, or a great contraction of the capillaries of the lungs caused by muscarin, will also result in dyspnœa and suffocation, and yet the lumen of the trachea is patent. As a further example: The saying, "The rain soaks the ground," cannot be assumed as implying "when the ground is wet it must have rained." The wetness of the ground may also be due to a rising of the soil-moisture, to the overflowing of a pool or to other causes. The saying, on the other hand, that cold, that is, loss of warmth, causes a .change in the consistency of water, and changes the fluid water into the solid ice, is an absolute one. When ice forms, cold must have been present in order to cause the change.

There exist but few absolute inclusive truths, and the conclusion that micro-organisms cause inflammation and suppuration does not belong in this category; inflammation and suppuration may follow on other causes than microbes.

The assumption that inflammation and suppuration may be present in the absence of microbes and be due to an irritation of the sympathetic nerves, explains how genuine inflammation and suppuration occur in entirely closed cavities, for the microbes could only reach these cavities by way of the blood-stream, and such a hypothesis is a difficult one to accept. When, however, in the pus of idiopathic meningitis, pleuritis, peritonitis and osteomyelitis micro-organisms are found, then these have either reached the closed cavity in the blood-stream or the micro-organisms have arisen within these cavities without getting there from the outside; or, finally, the small corpuscular bodies found are not true micro-organisms, but are the smallest possible particles of tissue, detritus, so to speak, which only in appearance resemble micro-organisms.

Neither of these three hypotheses can entirely satisfy us. Thousands of observations teach us that in the blood of healthy men neither micro-organisms nor their germs exist. We cannot say when, for example, a healthy individual slips on the ice and only splinters the tibia or bruises the skin and then suffers from a severe osteomyelitis, that the microbes have been carried by the blood-stream to the tibia and there have found a *locus minoris resistentiæ* and developed.

As to the view that microbes develop at the spot, all the evidence against the theory of a spontaneous generation speak. Although this theory cannot be absolutely negatived and banished, still it cannot be so frequently called upon as the frequency of idiopathic meningitis, pleuritis, peritonitis, osteomyelitis, etc., necessitates.

The third theory, that the corpuscular elements found in pus are not organisms, are not microbes, but the smallest possible particles of tissue detritus, remains still to be proved. On this question more light will be thrown when we speak of inoculation and transference of micro-organisms.

So much is proved that, aside from micro-organisms, still other irritants of the sympathetic nerves may cause abnormal action and lead to disturbances of nutrition which we call inflammation and suppuration.

What Demands will an Antiseptic satisfy in the Future?

The views just expressed give to the question of antiseptics an entirely different aspect. We do not exclusively require that antiseptics should have bactericide properties; we require only that they should protect the sympathetic nerves against abnormal irritation, or else that they should make these nerves unimpressionable.

According to this view the iodoform controversy seems useless. If iodoform is a drug which can render the sympathetic nerves unimpressionable to certain irritants, then will its healing power, its ability to check suppuration, its antitubercular property be clear, even though it lacks all bactericide action.

There are doubtless many other drugs and agents which have no further action on bacteria, and yet are most useful healing factors. Perhaps massage, perhaps irrigation of the field of operation are, in that they protect the sympathetic nerves against abnormal irritation and make them unimpressionable. This view explains why in pre-antiseptic times even so many wounds healed by first intention, and we find these methods in the older works on surgery laid down as assisting the healing of wounds. It is noteworthy, too, that in 1884, Lawson Tait reported 139 ovarian and parovarian cysts removed by laparotomy without a single death, although he did not use any antiseptic in these operations.

In these pages surgical wounds and diseases are chiefly treated of, but we must state that the theory of germs has also been applied to internal diseases and even earlier than to surgical. Tuberculosis, cholera, typhoid, croupous pneumonia, recurrent fever, malaria, gonorrhœa, syphilis, certain skin diseases, tetanus, etc., each has a supposititious micro-organism which causes the disease. Of the above diseases only the tubercle bacillus discovered by Koch, the cholera or comma bacillus, Obermayer's spiral bacillus, Neisser's gonococcus, are the unquestioned causes of tubercle, cholera, recurrent fever, and gonorrhœa. The assumption of a typhoid, malaria, and tetanus germ, as also that of croupous pneumonia and of syphilis, while plausible is not yet proved, and daily we see physicians in search of the germs of other diseases.

I would here remark that in internal medicine also the majority of logical deductions are not absolute.

Even in case of tuberculosis and of cholera, which unquestionably may be produced by the tubercle and comma bacillus respectively, we must grant the possibility of origin in another way than through these bacilli.

For each of the infectious diseases without exception there is supposed to be a bacillus, but it has only been determined for a relatively small number; even though, however, we knew the bacillus of each disease, we would not therefore have acquired as yet any assistance in the therapeusis of these diseases.

We are able to prevent wound diseases by an antiseptic operation and by antiseptic dressings, since thus we shut off the natural and only mode of entrance into the wound. In internal diseases, of bacillary origin, the manner of entrance of the bacilli is not known. They may enter the body through the lungs during respiration, by the intestinal tract, by an insignificant abrasion of the skin. We cannot, therefore, prevent their entrance into the body.

In case, however, pathogenetic microbes have gained entrance into the body, then is it more difficult to kill them than when in a wound. The internal use of bactericide agents is in its working very unreliable and occasionally injurious to the body. Cantani has suggested as a method of treatment of bacillary diseases the inoculation of material not dangerous to man in order to kill or render harmless the pathogenetic bacteria. As long, however, as a genus bacteriophagus is unknown such a proposition must remain therapeutically useless. We must still be satisfied, even as in the pre-bacteria age, with the control of single symptoms.

The Dawn of a New Era, which will have Greater Influence on Medicine than Bacteriology.

I will not pursue this question further, far exceeding as it does the limits of my paper, since we are on the threshold of a new era, when our views will suffer an essential change. The facts we are going to note will exert a far greater influence on physiology and pathology than has the doctrine of bacteria.

I will not theorize, but will stand firmly on the basis of observation and of fact, stating the consequences which may result.

At present we agree that blood consists of blood-serum and of three corpuscular elements—the red corpuscles, the leucocytes (the white blood corpuscles), and the hæmatoblasts.

The red corpuscles are the carriers of oxygen; when they come in contact with the muscles, glands and nerves, they give up their oxygen and take away the carbonic dioxide, and are the most essential sustainers of life and of tissue interchange. The hæmatoblasts constitute the coagulating property of the blood outside the body; and in the vessels, after ligation, they form the thrombus.

The leucocytes are granted varying functions, among others that of yielding the material of formation of the red corpuscles.

What action these leucocytes play in pus-formation we have already noted. They are granted an active part in the growth of tumors and in acute inflammations.

This glance at the composition of the blood shows us the groundwork of the physiology of to-day, and is the Ariadne-thread which leads us along the dark labyrinth of pathology. In the past few months the foundations of physiology have been shattered and the thread has been cut.

A. Mosso, who has carefully studied the blood of amphibia, birds, and man, by maceration of the blood in gastric juice, reached the same result as Rollet and Wooldridge, that the red corpuscles consist in an external envelope, in a fibrillary granular substance, and in a nucleus. The nucleus lies in the middle, and with tuft-like projections holds the external envelope fast; by the swelling of this envelope the insertion points of the nucleus look funnel-shaped. Between the envelope and the nucleus a layer is seen which consists of at least two porous substances which normally are homogeneous, but through change in the blood corpuscles this layer separates into two parts, a transparent and a yellowish hæmoglobin which also contains a slightly granular substance.

The red blood corpuscles change most readily, so that special care and expertness is needed to see an unaltered one under the microscope. Even disturbance by the object glass will alter them. This changeability varies with the animal and under the influence of different reagents. Even in the same animal corpuscles of varying strength and power of change are found. The stronger far outnumber the weaker. The difference in proportion between these two speaks for the strength and constitution of the animal.

The changes of the red blood corpuscles are manifold and up to now have been overlooked; and yet not overlooked, for they have been carefully watched and described, but the inferences have been false. In case of such sensitive and changeable bodies as the red corpuscles, the experiment of Cohnheim of stretching the mesentery of a frog under the microscope necessarily leads to error. Diapedesis affects readily and frequently the red corpuscles, the white less so.

The coagulation of the blood outside the body and in the vessels is only the consequence of the changes of the red corpuscles—that is to say, those which have the least resisting power, which break up into hæmatoblasts (Hayem, Bizzozero). Frequently enough in the coagulum or the thrombus strong, unaltered red corpuscles are found included.

A further change in the red blood corpuscles is a swelling, loss of color and formation within them of small and coarse granules; another step in the change consists in a translucency of the envelope of the swollen corpuscles, and at times we may witness a linear division. White blood corpuscles, pus corpuscles, and hæmatoblasts do not have any special shape, they are only altered red blood corpuscles. The corpuscles seen in pus are only changed red corpuscles which have migrated.

The changes of the blood corpuscles are not to be considered as stages of growth, of life, but as a death, a necrobiosis.

We may recognize the changes in strength of the blood corpuscles and the degree of their limit of life.

Healthy, unchanged red blood corpuscles cannot be colored, while all altered blood corpuscles according to the degree of change may be colored red in an eosin solution, 1 to 1000.

When the blood is defibrinated only the weaker corpuscles die and break up into hæmatoblasts, while in the defibrinated blood the strong corpuscles remain unchanged. Still the latter do not always remain unchanged. Babington claims that in oil, and E. Freund that in vaselin, the blood does not coagulate; Mosso says, however, that both oil and vaselin only retard coagulation.

When the blood is directly transferred from the carotid of a dog to the abdominal cavity of a fowl, or when defibrinated human blood is injected into the abdominaı cavity of a fowl, or a drop is placed in the anterior chamber of the eye of a puppy, we note, although the procedures were strictly antiseptic, changes in the individual blood corpuscles, as though microparasites had gained entrance to them.

Mosso has determined from his researches that the phagocytes described by Metschnikoff, that the changes in leukæmic blood noted by Virchow, that the bacillary alterations of typhoid-fever blood reported by Eichhorst, that the changes in the blood of cancer patients determined by Sappey, that the microbe wandering in the blood of malarial patients which Marchiafava and Celli found, that these and other changes were due to a necrobiosis of entirely normal red blood corpuscles.

It must also be especially noted that Mosso is able to determine the age of the corpuscular bodies found in pus. The youngest are the colored and swollen blood corpuscles; as these grow older they become larger, finely granulated; later they are grayish, and then very large, hyalin, in which latter state they remain in the capillaries of the lungs, liver, etc., and disappear from the circulation.

These observations of Mosso's are in accord with those of C. Heitzmann, of New York, published in 1883, in his microscopical morphology. Heitzmann's views when published received much comment and adverse criticism, but Mosso's corroboration gives strength to their great practical value.

Heitzmann says: "For a number of years I have noticed that the elements which are found in catarrhal lung affections and in tuberculosis in its acute and chronic form, were very pale and finely granular. Later I determined that the decolored blood and pus corpuscles of strong men were coarsely granular.

"By a microscopical examination of the blood I am able to determine the constitution of any individual without knowing anything about him or his manner of life.

"Points of value may be deduced from the difference in structure of the colorless blood corpuscles and from other considerations. For instance, the number of colorless blood corpuscles in a drop of blood varies greatly with the individual, and in general it holds that these corpuscles are the more scanty in number the better the constitution. A sleepless night, further, suffices to increase them, and from this fact I have often in jest been able to tell physicians after an examination of their blood as to whether their practice was lively or not, for in the former event sleepless nights or the demands of, and anxiety about patients were at work.

"Catarrhal inflammations of the mucous membrane also cause an increase in the number of colorless blood corpuscles, and a chronic inflammatory condition carries with it an undermined constitution. The red blood corpuscles are in color differently pronounced in different individuals; the paler the color the more certain the presence of pallor of the face or of chlorosis.

"The red blood corpuscles only run together in rollers when the serum contains a large amount of fibrin; in the blood of individuals in poor health the rouleaux are not found.   In individuals of mean strength they are sometimes present and again they are absent.

"In individuals of poor constitution, who had just passed through a serious disease, I found as a rule as well coarse as fine granular colorless blood corpuscles, as also in originally healthy individuals attacked by some chronic affection.

"Indeed the microscope tells us so much in regard to the health of man, that we cannot dispense with it any more than with the routine physical examination.

"Many years of observation have taught me the truth of this.

"The difference in appearance of living matter varies with the differences in individual constitution.   When in the urine, in the sputum, etc., pus corpuscles, or in a drop of blood colorless blood corpuscles, are found peculiar in one or another manner, then may the diagnosis of the individual constitution be made with certainty.

"When pus corpuscles resemble *a, b,* and *c* in the annexed figure, this is a sign of an aggravated tubercular or phthisical constitution.

"If pus and blood corpuscles like *d, e,* and *f,* are mingled with those like *g, h, k,* and *l, m, n,* then the inference is that a previously healthy constitution has become enfeebled by disease, and this the more the number of corpuscles resemble *a, b,* and *c.*

"Men of mean constitution when affected by chronic disease, or by factors which depress nutrition, have corpuscles like *l, m, n,* mixed with *a, b, c.*

"The presence of bodies like *a, b, c,* points only seldom and under the most favorable conditions to a long life; the more frequent the body *c,* the more certain it is that the end of the individual is near."

Mosso's observations, according to which pus corpuscles, the amœboid changes of the leucocytes, etc., are only red blood corpuscles changed in form, and are only different stages of disease and of death of the bioplasma of the red blood corpuscles—or, in other words, all the morphological elements found in the blood, in the lymph and in pus are only different degrees of the necrobiosis of the red blood corpuscles—these observations agree in every respect with Heitzmann's, and are pregnant of great practical value. The careful microscopic examination of the blood and pus is possibly for the practical physician and surgeon even as valuable from the stand-point of diagnosis and of prognosis as the determination of the tubercle-bacillus, the streptococcus, etc.

For examination of the blood a dear immersion lens is not necessary, nor an Abbe condenser, no coloring of the preparation, etc., but only the routine method and an ordinary microscope such as was used in the pre-bacterial era.

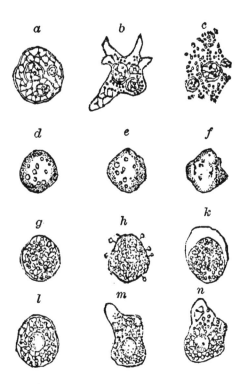

From the corroborative experiments of Mosso and of Heitzmann it follows that the blood and lymph corpuscles are very sensitive and changeable organisms, and that slight irritations, such as a current of atmospheric air, disturbance by the object glass, etc., are sufficient to kill or alter them.

Among the irritations affecting the blood corpuscles those due to the action of microbes play a prominent *rôle;* but it is one-sided to ignore all other irritants acting on the blood and the lymph corpuscles, and to lay the chief blame on the microbes. With the knowledge of the different kinds of irritants,

however, our understanding of disease processes has not increased; as long as we do not have a more exact knowledge
of the different qualities which the protoplasm of the blood
and of the lymph corpuscles suffer as the result of the action
of various irritants, so long will the physiological and pathological processes taking place in the animal body remain in
darkness.   Here the ax is to be laid, and the way cut through
which the light of observation may shine to disperse the
darkness surrounding this question.

In case of the organs of sense the question is a relatively
simple one, for the different irritants act in the same way.   On
the primary radicles of the optic nerve irritants cause only
sensation of light.   On the acoustic nerve different irritants
only cause sensations of sound; on the gustatory and the tac-
tile nerves the effects of all irritants are taste and sensation.
Far different are the results on the single cells of the animal
body, where different qualities of irritation cause different
changes and movements of the irritated cells.   A few examples will clear this.

Cienkowski has made some very interesting observations
on certain monads in this connection.   The vampyrella spiro-
gyrà is a small, microscopic, reddish, structureless amœba,
which of all the water plants seeks only a certain alga, the
spirogyra, as food, rejecting all others.   It finds a spirogyra,
sucks its contents, seeks another, and repeats the process.
Other algæ, such as vaucheria, œdogonia, it rejects.

Cienkowski noticed the same behavior on the part of another monad.   The colpodella pugnax feeds only on the chla-
mydomonas, seeks it and after sucking out the contents seeks
another to repeat the process.

Now no one will claim that these monads act from choice;
the processes are simple, the result of special irritants.   The
spirogyra affects the vampyrella, even as does the chlamydo-
monas the colpodella, and these monads are attracted to the
action as it were.

But why wander so far when we can find far more convincing examples in our own bodies.

We know that the intestinal wall is covered by epithelial
cells, that each epithelial cell is an independent organism, a
living being, so to speak, with developed functions, which, even
as the amœbæ and rhizopods, takes nourishment by active con-

traction, assimilates this and rejects what is not suitable. It has long been known that the mono-cellular being selects for its nourishment what is beneficial to it and rejects what is harmful or useless. We know that the intestinal epithelium has the property of selecting the fat drops from food, and of utilizing them later in the radicles of the chyle vessels.

The epithelial cell, further, selects the nourishment suitable for itself even as does the vampyrella. If fat drops and minute particles of pigment reach it, it selects the former and rejects the latter. We may even go further. In the digestion of albuminate by peptone a great variety of material in soluble form results—for instance ptomaïnes—which is not absorbed by the normal epithelium of the intestines.

Still more interesting is the property of the epithelial cell in the different glands; it takes certain material from the blood and neglects other material; the portion acquired having become broken up and altered, a portion of the new product passes through the efferent duct of the gland, and a portion returns to the lymph and the blood current.

The same process occurs in the tissue elements of the parenchyma of the glands, as, for example, in the liver. The products of digestion reach the liver through the vena porta; the glandular cells of the organ separate these products, and thus altered they are returned to the circulation. True enough portions injurious to the organism are emptied into the duodenum, and without entering the circulation, make the circuit a number of times from the intestines through the vena porta to the liver and again into the intestine until they are finally passed with the fæces; other material, such as an excess of sugar, is converted into glycogen in the liver and returned to the blood as needed, and this wonderful property of the epithelial and gland cells is only the result of irritation of living protoplasm.

Protoplasm, blood corpuscles, lymph and gland cells may become diseased, may be more or less sensitive to irritants. The partial or total disease of the red plasma results, then, in a partial or total disease of the organism. These small living principles, the blood, lymph, epithelial and gland cells are microbes, the biology of which remains still to be determined. Only when we have laid the groundwork, thoroughly sifted the essence, cause and quality, in short the causality of the irritability of the protoplasm, only then will we determine from every stand-point the vitality, the life principle, the life strength.

We must, however, yield to no illusion. Owing to the limitations of our senses and the incompleteness of our methods of research, we cannot hope soon to solve the problem; we must ever be careful not to err in the final result. It is to be hoped that, by following out the road opened by Mosso and Heitzmann, by applying their tests to all elementary cells of the living organism, we may reach a soil containing in its depths rich biological truths, which need only be laid bare by careful and constant work. To all vigorous, unprejudiced workers in this soil I would say God speed!